Ethical Dilemmas in Health Promotion

Ethical Dilemmas in Health Promotion

Editor

SPYROS DOXIADIS
President, Foundation for Research in Childhood, Athens

Editorial Committee:

Roger Blaney
Senior Lecturer, Department of Community Medicine, Queen's University, Belfast

Alastair Campbell
Professor of Christian Ethics and Practical Theology, New College, University of Edinburgh, Edinburgh

Heleen M Dupuis
Professor of Ethics, Faculty of Medicine, Leiden University, Leiden

Lucien Karhausen
Officer of the Commission of the EEC, Brussels

Susie Stewart
Technical Editor, Glasgow

A Wiley Medical Publication

JOHN WILEY & SONS
Chichester · New York · Brisbane · Toronto · Singapore

Reprinted May 1990

British Library Cataloguing in Publication Data:

Ethical Dilemmas in Health Promotion
1. Public health—Moral and ethical aspects
I. Doxiadis, Spyros II. Blaney, Roger
174′.2 RA427

ISBN 0 471 91313 8

Library of Congress Cataloging-in-Publication Data:

Ethical Dilemmas in Health Promotion
(A Wiley medical publication)
1. Public health—Moral and ethical aspects.
2. Health promotion—Moral and ethical aspects.
3. Medicine, Preventive—Moral and ethical aspects.
4. Medical ethics. I. Doxiadis, Spyros. II. Blaney, R. (Roger) III. Series [DNLM:
1. Ethics, Medical. 2. Public Health. WA 100 I34]
RA427.25.I47 1987 174′.2 86-24573

ISBN 0 471 91313 8

Printed and bound in Great Britain by
Biddles Ltd, Guildford and King's Lynn

Contents

Preface

My first thoughts on the need to study the ethical problems in the field of health promotion and disease prevention arose in my mind when I was Minister of Health in Greece. My initiative and planning for various new public health projects, such as extensive health education and fluoridation of water made me consider, not in theory but in actual practice, the responsibilities and rights of the state in attempting, for example, to change the life-style of citizens or to add a chemical substance to the drinking water.

So, when my term as Minister came to an end, I started to explore the possibility of a multidisciplinary study of the various ethical and moral dilemmas that arise in all efforts to promote public health. I wrote to various friends, I received an enthusiastic and interested response and four years ago I started planning this project. I approached Professor Edward Bennett, Director of Health and Safety of the Commission of the European Communities and my plans received the approval of the Panel of Social Medicine and Epidemiology of the EEC under the Chairmanship of Professor Walter W. Holland. The Panel appointed Roger Blaney and Lucien Karhausen as members of a small planning team. To this team, which developed into the present Editorial Committee, Heleen Dupuis, Alastair Campbell, and Susie Stewart as Technical Editor were subsequently added.

We started collecting a team of experts from many disciplines and we had the first meeting of all the participants in the project at a workshop in Athens in January 1985, sponsored by NATO Science Council. The proceedings of this workshop were published in 1985 by Martinus Nijhoff, Dordrecht under the title of *Ethical Issues in Preventive Medicine*. At that meeting we agreed to produce a book on *Ethical Dilemmas in Health Promotion* to explore in more detail the many issues raised in the Athens workshop. The Editorial Committee has met on numerous occasions since then and we also had a meeting of all the authors in Luxembourg for another exchange of views and comments on individual chapters. We decided to confine ourselves mainly to ethical issues in preventive medicine and health promotion in the developed countries of which we have direct personal experience. The problems and practice of prevention in the developing countries are of great importance but they are very different and beyond the scope of this book. So, after another round of meetings of the Editorial Committee, mainly to avoid repetitions and overlapping, we finished the work.

I would like to thank Professor Edward Bennett and Professor Walter Holland for their encouragement, and the Directorate-General of Employment, Social Affairs and Education of the Commission of the European Communities for financial support. The Foundation for Research in Childhood in Athens has provided all administrative and organizational services and has also contributed significantly to the cost of the whole project, and for this help I am particularly grateful.

I also wish to thank most warmly all the authors for their contributions and for their willingness to work with us with great patience, and above all I wish to express my gratitude to the members of the Editorial Committee for their hard work and friendly cooperation. Finally, I would like to thank John Jarvis and his associates at John Wiley and Sons for their help and expertise in the production of the book.

SPYROS DOXIADIS

List of Contributors

DAN E. BEAUCHAMP *Professor of Health Policy and Administration and Professor of Social and Administrative Medicine, School of Public Health, The University of North Carolina at Chapel Hill, 263 Rosenau Building, 201 Chapel Hill, North Carolina 27514–6201, USA*

ROGER BLANEY *Senior Lecturer and Acting Head of Department, Department of Community Medicine, Institute of Clinical Science, The Queen's University of Belfast, Grosvenor Road, Belfast BT12 6BJ, Northern Ireland*

MARTINE BUNGENER *Economist, LEGOS, Université de Paris IX Dauphine, Place du M^{al} de Lattre de Tassigny, 75016 Paris, France*

ALASTAIR V. CAMPBELL *Professor of Christian Ethics and Practical Theology, University of Edinburgh, New College, The Mound, Edinburgh EH1 2LX, Scotland*

SPYROS DOXIADIS *Professor and President, Foundation for Research in Childhood, 42 Amalias Street, Athens 105 58, Greece*

G. R. DUNSTAN *Emeritus Professor of Moral and Social Theology, University of London and Honorary Research Fellow, Department of Theology, University of Exeter, Queen's Building, The University, Exeter EX4 4QH, England*

HELEEN M. DUPUIS *Professor of Ethics, METAMEDICA, Faculty of Medicine, p/a Pathologisch Laboratorium, Rijksuniversiteit Leiden, Postbus 9603, 2300 RC Leiden, The Netherlands*

LEON EISENBERG *Professor and Chairman, Department of Social Medicine and Health Policy, Harvard Medical School, 25 Shattuck Street, Boston, Massachussetts 02115, USA*

OLIVIER JEANNERET *Professor and Head, Institute of Social and Preventive Medicine, University of Geneva, 27 Quai Charles-Page, CH-1211 Geneva 4, Switzerland*

LUCIEN KARHAUSEN *Officer of the Commission of the European Communities, Directorate of Health and Safety, Bâtiment Jean Monnet, Plâteau du Kirchberg, L-2920 Luxembourg*

A. H. M. KERKHOFF *Director, Public Health Services, Warmonderweg 3, 2334 AA Leiden, The Netherlands*

E. G. KNOX *Professor, Health Services Research Centre, Department of Social Medicine, The Medical School, Edgbaston, Birmingham B15 2TJ, England*

M. MANCIAUX *Professor of Public Health, Nancy University, BP 184, F-50405 Vandoeuvre, France*

JEAN MARTIN *Lecturer in Social and Preventive Medicine, Institute of Social and Preventive Medicine, Bugnon 17, CH-1005, Lausanne, Switzerland*

GENEVIEVE PINET *Regional Officer for Health Legislation, World Health Organization, 8 Scherfigsvej, DK-2100 Copenhagen, Denmark*

SIR EDWARD POCHIN *Physician, National Radiological Protection Board, Chilton Didcot, Oxfordshire OX11 0RQ, England*

LUC RAYMOND *Senior Research Fellow, Department of Social and Preventive Medicine, University of Geneva, 27 Quai Charles-Page, CH-1211 Geneva 4, Switzerland*

CLAIRE RAYNER *Nurse, Journalist, Holly Wood House, Roxborough Avenue, Harrow-on-the-Hill, Middlesex HO1 3BU, England*

POVL RIIS *Professor of Internal Medicine, University of Copenhagen, Medical-Gastroenterological Department C, Herlev University Hospital, DK-2730 Herlev, Denmark*

ALFRED SAND *Professor of Public Health, Université Libre de Bruxelles Campus Erasme 595, B-1070 Brussels, Belgium*

TOMA STRASSER *Senior Lecturer, Department of Social and Preventive Medicine, University of Geneva, 27 Quai Charles-Page, CH-1211 Geneva 4, Switzerland*

Introduction

SPYROS DOXIADIS

> 'We must start from what is known. But things are known in two senses : known to us and known absolutely. Presumably we must start from what is known to *us*.' (Aristotle Ethics. Book one.)

At the end of World War 2 the discovery of the inhuman experiments by doctors on prisoners of war and detainees and the Nuremberg trials opened a new era in the long history of medical ethics. The first step, the immediate result of the trials, was the formulation of what has been called the Nuremberg Code (1947) which was in fact part of a sentence issued in the case of the United States versus Karl Brandt. Similar codes adding to and improving the code have since been formulated, mainly at the initiative of the World Medical Association and of the World Health Organization.

As a reaction also to the totalitarian principles of the dictatorships during and after World War 2 and because of the extension of education to larger numbers of people, a new awareness has developed of the rights of the individual and of the obligation of the State to care for its citizens on the one hand and to respect their autonomy on the other. And this awareness has gradually spread to include the rights of the individual not only against political oppression but also against the paternalism exhibited by professions such as law, religion and medicine. The practitioners of these professions, perhaps most notably the physicians, began to realize that they could no longer be the sole judges in matters of life and death. They needed the help of other professions and disciplines and they needed the understanding and the cooperation of patients and their families.

These developments resulted in a large number of discussions and publications around the broad subject of medical ethics. Special centres of medical ethics were created, special societies were founded and some philosophers, ethicists and physicians devoted most of their scientific work to the subject.

Not surprisingly, most of these activities focussed at first on ethical problems arising out of treatment in the one-to-one doctor to patient relationship that is the norm of medical practice. Doctors, patients, and the public in general have always preferred short-term satisfaction and immediate results to long-term social benefits. But in the last few years it has become clear that in matters related to health the ethical dilemmas in therapeutic medicine are not the only ones that give rise to concern. The realization that, in spite of new methods of treating the main killing diseases, there are limits to the ability of medicine to restore health and that therefore more emphasis should be given to prevention, has led to the conclusion that ethical issues in health promotion, health care and disease prevention deserve special attention.

The ethical problems in the traditional preventive medicine concerned with infectious diseases did not seem so great since public health, state intervention and individual measures produced full benefits with very little cost. However, since most of our major health problems now relate to environmental and behavioural factors, some of the greatest obstacles to progress in this field appear to be not only in the question of individual rights but in other issues such as cost including loss of jobs. The reduction in tobacco consumption, for example, may lead to unemployment in some sectors of agriculture and industry. The benefits to society from nuclear power, such as cheap electricity, expansion of industry with more jobs available, are to be measured against the health risks arising from this development.

Another factor creating new problems is the increasing awareness of large sections of the public of the possibilities of modern medicine and the resulting expectation and demand from the state and from the medical profession for better health services.

Finally, the increasing cost of medicine and of health services has created another group of dilemmas in the priorities for the allocation of scarce resources.

All the above developments in the fields of health promotion and disease prevention have created new ethical problems very different from those of therapeutic medicine but of at least equal importance.

Six important differences between therapeutic and preventive medicine from an ethical point of view can be identified.

Firstly, in therapeutic medicine, one person or a small number of people present the health problem. In preventive medicine much larger numbers are involved. An unethical decision would, therefore, affect many more people.

Secondly, in therapeutic medicine, the person or persons are ill when they present with the problem. But, particularly in primary prevention, the subjects are usually healthy. Unethical decisions will therefore affect people who have been previously entirely or apparently healthy.

Thirdly, the responsibility in therapeutic medicine is usually vested in one doctor or a small number of doctors or other health professionals. In this context, the responsibility of the state for ethical matters as distinct from legal responsibility is very remote. In preventive medicine, on the other hand, the direct responsibility of the state is often considerable. But the community physician or health planner is rarely in individual contact with the subject of his work and may therefore feel less responsible for his decisions. The problem of abortion, of euthanasia, of the mentally defective newborn presented in a clinical situation with an individual patient will appear very different from a consideration of similar problems in a large anonymous population. Furthermore there can be great danger when 'systems' make decisions.

Fourthly, in therapeutic medicine, the results of a decision are usually assessed within a few days, weeks, or months of consultation. The results of decisions in preventive medicine frequently take a much longer time to evaluate. Again the responsibility is remote, and it may, therefore, tend to be forgotten.

Fifthly, in therapeutic medicine, the criteria of success or failure are easily defined—death or life, an additional life or not, interruption of pregnancy or not, transplantation or not. In preventive medicine, the criteria of success or failure are defined much less easily or clearly because there are so many factors involved. Here again, this complexity of aetiological or contributing factors may tend to lessen the feeling of responsibility in those making the decisions.

Lastly, while decisions in therapeutic medicine are usually independent of the cultural, social and economic background of the subject, many decisions in preventive medicine affect disadvantaged groups with inadequate knowledge of their own rights and of the consequences of possible courses of action. Our responsibility to protect the rights of such groups is great. In an undernourished population, for example, the manifestation causing most concern among parents is blindness of their children caused by vitamin A deficiency. This can be prevented by administration of some vitamin drops, a relatively easy and cheap measure, which will satisfy the parents. But this result may blunt their sensitivity to the more difficult and equally serious problem of undernutrition and may also provoke among the administrators or other groups able to help a feeling of false satisfaction and therefore lead to inertia.

As the title of our book *Ethical Dilemmas in Health Promotion* shows, our objective was to explore the ethical issues arising in all projects, great or small, by the state or by agencies or by individuals, aiming at preventing disease and promoting health.

It is natural that such a subject should involve a multidisciplinary approach because health care, health promotion, disease prevention and ethics encompass many disciplines. Almost all authors have had much experience in their fields and are in daily contact with the problems they describe and analyse.

Since this book is aimed at a large audience composed not only of medical and public health practitioners, but of other health professions and many related disciplines as well, the first part, entitled 'Theoretical Background', contains five chapters which seek to examine ethical theory and terminology, to highlight the main conflict between autonomy and the common good, and to trace the evolution of medical ethics and of our concepts of disease prevention.

In the second part, entitled 'Policies and General Problems', the emphasis is on theoretical and practical problems directly related to policies and practice. Among aspects examined are the conflict between public and individual interests, paternalism, the need to abandon fundamentalism in medical ethics, the strengths and limitations of health legislation, health economics and ethics, value conflicts in health promotion policies, and estimation of occupational risk.

The third part deals with 'Specific Issues' and covers ethical aspects of reproductive medicine, child health, screening programmes and prevention trials. There is also a chapter on the organization of ethical control and one on the role of the mass communication media in health education.

This subject of ethical dilemmas in public health and preventive medicine is a very difficult and complex one. In the final chapter of the book, I have attempted to draw some conclusions from preceding contributions, to make some recommendations for the future, and to stress above all the importance of alerting as wide an audience as possible—the general public, individual practitioners, private and government bodies, academic institutions, decision-makers, legislators—to these ethical issues which confront us all.

PART A
THEORETICAL BACKGROUND

Ethical Dilemmas in Health Promotion
Edited by S. Doxiadis

CHAPTER 1

Evolution and Mutation in Medical Ethics

G. R. DUNSTAN

SUMMARY

The purpose of this chapter is to trace developments in medical ethics since the Second World War. These have occurred partly as a necessary consequence of developments in medical science and technology and partly in reaction from totalitarian violations of human liberties and dignity. The developments discussed are mostly those formulated in the major Codes and Declarations adopted for international observance since that of Nuremberg in 1947. Medical ethics as such is distinguished from the more complicated ethics of 'health care'. In the language of ethics, care is taken to limit the unreflecting use of the rhetoric of 'rights'. The primary purpose of an ethics of medicine is to delineate good practice. This purpose can be, and sometimes is, obscured by philosophical analysis unrelated to practice, and by legal complication governed by litigious interest and intent. And since ethics embodies mutual expectation, attention should now be focussed on the ethical obligations of patients to match those which they expect from their practitioners.

INTRODUCTION

No civilization can exist without an ethics, a pattern of mutual expectations and obligations. These are grounded in tradition, in historical continuity from a distant past. Medical ethics stands thus in Western civilization, with an ancestry traced back through Christian, Jewish and Arabic cultures to the Greeks and, behind them, to the ancient civilizations of the Middle East, Egyptian, Babylonian, Hittite, Assyrian. Throughout them all, the moral obligations attending medical practice—which is what 'medical ethics' means—have been shaped by religion (sometimes compounded with astrology and magic), philosophy and social and political control.

Yet into continuity there erupts from time to time a radical discontinuity, a mutation in what looked like steady evolution. We live in such a period of change today. The process is sometimes called a 'revolution'. But words with evocative and ambiguous overtones are better avoided in ethical discussion. It has been occasioned partly by changes in the knowledge-base of medicine itself, medical science, creating a new medical technology and new, penetrating opportunities for medical practice. And since one phase in these developments coincided with the emergence of a particularly ruthless political tyranny, the Nazi regime in Germany, they were exploited in ways which, once revealed, shocked the world and set off waves of fear which dominate discussion still: in popular debate the cheapest substitute for reasoned objection to a new practice is the jibe, 'back to the Nazis' or 'back to Belsen'. The man in the white coat is made an object of fear. Even with peaceful, benign intent, technology can dominate; its expensive professional and bureaucratic management can overwhelm.

In reaction, then, to political tyranny and to the feeling of corporate domination there comes an upsurge of libertarian sentiment; it is particularly strong at present in the USA. It finds voice in the language of rights, amplified by consumerism. Upon a traditional ethics of professional obligation there is imposed an ethics of adversarial external control. And since one weapon of consumerism is litigation, in resort to the courts for redress for every wrong, real or imagined, medical ethics becomes, in some quarters, a counter in the gambles of the law. 'Ethical' becomes that which will give a physician a successful defence to an action; 'unethical' becomes that which will cost him or his insurers heavy damages. From this results defensive medicine, a practice overshadowed by fear. This is the environment in response to which an evolving medical ethics, in the late twentieth century, is undergoing mutation.

A new dimension is opened by the language of 'health care'. 'Medical ethics', as traditionally used, implies 'the obligations of a moral nature which govern the practice of medicine'.[1] As such it has referred to practitioners corporately, in their brotherhood, or craft guild, or, now, as a profession. An 'ethics of health care' envisages a wider community. It presupposes a highly complex modern state, organizing provision for its citizens' health. The issues deemed ethical now range more widely. They cover the provision of services and care, whether by the state or by private practitioners and commercially owned hospitals and paid for by private insurance or by both systems together. They call for political decisions regarding the allocation of resources as to research, or to primary or routine health care, or to expensive innovative therapies, or to the aged, or the young, or the handicapped, or the socially deprived; or to health education and preventive medicine. Medicine is seen as a factor in social policy and therefore in political debate; and inevitably the economy and ethics of the pharmaceutical industry become involved. The change from 'medical ethics' to 'the ethics of health care' is not, therefore, simply a change of language;

it indicates a wider subject. This chapter will confine itself to the first, the narrower, while not unaware of the second.

A moment's reflection will determine why this should be so. It were folly to attempt to delineate 'the ethics of health care'—intellectually either arrogant or inept, practically useless. Each discrete element in the promotion of health care has its own ethics—or most of them have; other chapters in this book examine some of them, and even so there are gaps. Politics has its ethics. The allocation of national resources to fund national policies is ultimately a matter of political decision, and governments differ in their openness to persuasion. There are ethical and unethical ways of mounting political pressure, as members of health services realize when they decide for or against strike action to demonstrate their corporate will. Improvements in the environment—purer air, cleaner water, better housing, town planning and community development—contribute to health care. So do epidemiological studies, preventive vaccination and immunization, and imposed protective measures like the wearing of seat-belts in cars, the adding of fluoride to water supplies and the control of pesticides and of additives to food. Education for health includes elementary prophylaxis, an understanding of diet and nutrition, and dissuasion from the abuse of alcohol, tobacco, medicines and drugs. Each of these activities commands an ethics in its own right, and some are treated elsewhere in this volume. The practice of community medicine, and of industrial medicine, have ethical norms incorporating the ethics of medicine in general but developing others special to each discipline, concerned primarily as each is with whole populations or socio-economic groups. It would be, therefore, a vain pursuit to look for an ethical formulation to cover all these aspects of health care. This chapter will concentrate on the growth of the main stem of medical ethics in the last generation or so; other chapters may trace the lines of differentiated growth, or point to the buds from which growth has yet to develop.

ETHICS IN MEDICAL RESEARCH

One requirement in an ethics is that its expectations be known: we must know what to expect of one another in situations roughly comparable. So Codes of Practice have signalled the ethical judgments of this half-century.[2] They began with the Nuremberg Code of 1947. That Code embodied 10 principles upon which the Nuremberg Tribunal had given judgment upon 23 defendants, mostly physicians, accused of crimes involving experiments on human subjects. The principles governed the conduct of research, outlining the requirements of free consent, of the scientific validity and probable utility of the experiments, the protection of subjects from harm, and the balance of risk against the prospective beneficial outcome in terms of a worthwhile contribution to medical science unobtainable by other means.

The Code proved to be the basic draft for future work. The World Medical Association (WMA) amplified it in the Declaration of Helsinki, 1964, the text of which was fully revised in 1975 and again amended in 1983. After a preamble and statement of general principles, it distinguished between Medical Research Combined with Professional Care (Clinical Research) and Non-Therapeutic (or Non-Clinical) Biomedical Research, and drew rules accordingly. The distinction between 'therapeutic' and 'non-therapeutic' research, though useful within limits, was to dominate and sometimes to confuse subsequent ethical thinking—for often the distinction is too neat to match the facts of the case. What, for instance, of research procedures designed to gain knowledge of general validity but not to benefit particular patients, conducted incidentally as part of a therapeutic experimental procedure designed for the patient's good? Once it is established as axiomatic that a proxy consent may be given for an experimental or research procedure which may benefit a child, but that it may not be given for a procedure not designed directly for that child's potential benefit, all non-therapeutic research on children must cease; and this would hinder the gaining of knowledge about normal functioning which paediatricians may need to establish the criteria of abnormality. Some endemic diseases are specific to children, some fatal to them; others, like diarrhoea and malaria, affect children more seriously than adults. To establish causes and remedies for these, research with children is necessary. One significant addition made to the Helsinki Code in 1983 reflected increasing consideration for children: a minor child's consent, if obtainable, should be obtained, as well as that of his parent or guardian. A study and attempted resolution of ethical problems in relation to paediatric research has been published recently by the Institute of Medical Ethics in London.[3]

Emphasis on the necessity and ethical validity of research involving children, and especially in preventive medicine, is strong in the *Proposed International Guidelines for Biomedical Research Involving Human Subjects*, a joint project of the World Health Organization (WHO) and the Council for International Organizations of Medical Science (CIOMS) published in 1982.[4] It marks an evolutionary step beyond the Helsinki Declaration in that it goes beyond research in which subjects are envisaged as individuals, one by one, into community-based research, and that with strong prophylactic intent, particularly in developing countries where need is highest but input least. Public health policies, initiated and carried through by governments, are not exempt from ethical scrutiny, nor without need of ethical control.

Local guidelines for research have been published by national and professional bodies in different countries, following Nuremberg and Helsinki principles. The Medical Research Council (MRC) is one such body in England; its latest statement is a principled guide to practice in the use of personal medical information for purposes of research.[5] The National Commission for the Protection of Human Subjects of Biomedical and Behavioural Research is another such body in the USA. Disciplinary groups like the British Paediatric Association have issued codes for their members; the Association of the British Pharmaceutical Industry has issued a code for the conduct of clinical trials in medical general practice.

Such guidelines are followed by the Research Ethics Committees, or Ethical Review Boards, set up in association with hospitals or university centres of research to validate, or not, proposals for research involving human subjects. These committees include non-medical members, another new expression of the ethical mutation: members of the public, potential patients or subjects of research, are now involved with the scientists and practitioners in the ethical control of their undertakings. The process of lay supervision could be overdone to the point of the moral paralysis of the practitioner: if he were allowed no freedom of decision in anything that matters, having all decisions taken from him by a committee, court, or board—as some enthusiasts for citizen or consumer participation advocate—his professional standing, value and competence would vanish with his independence. The object of research ethics committees is to reconcile the claims of a proper zeal for research—for that disciplined and purposeful curiosity proper to science in all its forms—with public accountability and the protection of the vulnerable. The Royal College of Physicians of England, whose initiatives brought these committees into being, has, after some years of experience, issued guidelines for their constitution and practice.[6]

The safeguarding of confidences has been one solemn duty in medicine to which the epithet 'Hippocratic' is unfailingly applied; it has the highest ethical obligation. New technical developments, like computer technology in the storage of information, and new developments in professional cooperation in health care, have alike required reconsideration of the duty. Both in research and in clinical practice confidential information is handled by more people. Clearly, the obligation of secrecy must be shared by them corporately. Equally clearly, the interests of patients—children in danger of abuse, neglect or violence are one obvious group—must not be put at risk by a refusal to share information between colleagues, within the common obligation not improperly to disclose. Guidelines are being developed to meet this need. Among them is *The Confidentiality of Medical Records*, The Report of a Working Party of the Advisory Panel for Social Medicine and Epidemiology in the European Economic Community.[7]

PROTECTION OF HUMAN LIFE

At stake is the protection of the human person from harm; and the issues come most sharply into focus at the beginning and at the end of life. Two series of Declarations pertain. In 1948 the WMA attempted to re-write the so-called Hippocratic Oath in modern terms. This resulted in the Declaration of Geneva, which was revised again in 1968. It contained the statement, 'I will maintain the utmost respect for human life from the time of conception'. But advances since 1948 in embryology, and in the techniques of *in vitro* fertilization (IVF) brought even those simple words into confusion. 'When does human life begin?' is a biological question, though it is often posed as a moral question. The biologists can give no certain answer: sperm and oocyte have 'life' independently before their cells are fused in fertilization; not all products of the fertilization of human gametes are indisputably human; nuclear transfer and cellular manipulation can, in theory, and in dawning practice, derive mammalian progeny from unfertilized cells. So at Venice in October 1983 the WMA revised the Declaration of Geneva to take cognizance of this doubt. The 'time of conception' was amended to 'the time of its—that is, life's—beginning.'

Meanwhile the properly moral question is vigorously exercised: at what point in the development of the human embryo or fetus do or should we attribute to it such a moral status as to assure it the protection due to a human being? What, in consequence, are the ethics governing the fertilization of human oocytes specifically for observation and research—or governing this use of embryos left 'spare' after IVF and embryo replacement? Contemporary pressure groups, claiming dogmatic support from pronouncements of the Roman Catholic Church—echoed, indeed, in other Christian confessions—would claim absolute protection for the human being from the moment of fertilization.[8] But this is a novelty, dating only from Pope Pius IX in 1869. The Western tradition, including the Jewish, Christian and Islamic faiths, for between 3000 and 4000 years, has graded the protection *pari passu* with the growth of the fetus towards maturity.[9] How the question will be resolved is of great importance to medicine. Vast potential knowledge is locked up in the cleaving human embryo, if only embryologists and geneticists are allowed to work on it, as they claim that they can, without sacrifice of our beliefs about the essential value of human life. Benefits are predicted not only for the study of and medical attention to fertility and infertility, but also for related fields in immunology, the aetiology of congenital handicap and of neoplasms, and perhaps the eventual development of gene therapy to replace the reparative grafting of whole organs.[10,11] The issues are controversial enough to secure political attention. In Britain a Committee of Inquiry set up by the Government has reported.[12] It recommends the continuance of the research under strict licence and supervision, and it would set a term of 14 days from fertilization beyond which research on human embryos may not continue—a date consistent with some professional representations in Britain and the USA, but held by some to be needlessly restrictive—two or three days more could yield useful knowledge. Strong pressure groups would allow no research on human embryos at all. The Medical Research Council and the Royal College of Obstetricians and Gynaecologists have set up together a Voluntary Licensing Authority to supervise IVF and research on embryos in the United Kingdom, until Parliament can set up its own statutory body to do so.

Opposition to the research is the more strenuous by those already shocked at the growing resort to abortion for reasons beyond strict therapeutic necessity—beyond, that is, the safeguarding of the mother—including the avoidance of a pre-natally diagnosed, or statistically possible, congenital handicap. The WMA's Declaration of Oslo in 1970 reflected the conflict of views on the ethics of therapeutic abortion and gave very cautious guidance to doctors for their practice in countries where the law permits termination of pregnancy. But constant progress in medical science changes the conditions for the debate. More accurate diagnosis of handicap earlier in pregnancy gives counsellors and parents more reliable information on which to base a decision, with the option of earlier termination if they so decide. And some do so decide, and conceive again, and bear a healthy child—and so hand on the heterozygous or recessive gene to embarrass a later generation. Yet progress in that very research on cleaving embryos, which anti-abortion groups so determinedly oppose, may yet turn the edge of the question: if the defective gene or chromosomal pattern could be detected *in vitro* and, possibly some day, be corrected there, the crude resort to abortion—or the birth of a severely handicapped child—might in some instances be prevented. Our ethics are an interim ethics, evolving with evolving knowledge and practice.

A similar process is discernible in the ethics of terminal care and the medical association with death. For millennia the obvious signs of death, commonly and clinically observed, sufficed for most human purposes. They did not suffice when transplant surgery began to exert its demand for organs for grafting, tissue-compatible and still biologically functional. All human sentiment and justice require that the donor or source of cadaver organs be truly dead before they are removed; yet if removal is more than a little delayed, they are proportionately less useful for their purpose. The 'brainstem dead' patient, whose vital organs and tissues are kept functional by ventilation and pharmacological infusion, could prove to be the ideal source of organs for grafting. The critical task was to determine the fact of death, given the differential speeds at which organs and tissues cease to function. The general ethics were stated in a WMA Declaration of Sydney in 1968; the clinical criteria were laid down by the appropriate medical bodies, in Britain by a Working Party of all the Royal Colleges. But again, changing practice calls for a change in the Codes. The WMA, in 1968, invoked the electroencephalograph (EEG) as 'the most helpful' of diagnostic aids. At its meeting in Venice in 1983 the WMA deleted the reference to the EEG, because practice had moved beyond it. The Venice re-statement did, however, underline the importance of the death of the brainstem for related decisions.

Meanwhile another ethical surge in terminal care has concentrated attention on the dying patient in his own right, and not as a subject for research or as a source of donor tissues. The hospice movement has pioneered a new concept of care for the dying, combining the most advanced pharmacological aids in the control of pain and distress with sensitive attention to the spiritual, emotional and social needs of dying people and their families.[13] This too is in a phase of development. Having cultured (so to speak) its skills in hospices and units established for that purpose, it is now extending those skills into teaching and general hospitals and into community practice. And as the control of pain, and terminal care, improve, so the old ethical dilemmas of the euthanasia debate become obsolete: they point to a past which is slipping away. It is not necessary, given proper medical resources, to kill a patient to relieve his pain.

MEDICINE AND POLITICAL DURESS

Medical ethics have never evolved in isolation from their environment. Two other Declarations point, sadly, to the political environment in which medicine is practised and consciences are stretched. The Declaration of Tokyo in 1975 was promulgated to strengthen the position of doctors in countries where torture or other cruel, degrading or inhuman treatments are instruments of punishment or political control. It forbids their participation in all such. Yet the dilemma in some countries is real and acute. When torture, physical or psychological, is inflicted as an instrument of politics, or of policing or of military tactics, or when mutilation is carried out as a punishment for theft or other moral offence or crime, what is the doctor to do? A strict reading of the terms of the Declaration would oblige him to abstain from the whole enterprise, lest he appear to 'countenance, condone or participate' in it. Yet this would be to leave the victim in worse hands, to suffer more. The Declaration of Hawaii, 1977, issued by the World Psychiatric Association, was similarly designed to strengthen doctors in their refusal to countenance or support the abuse of psychiatry as an instrument of political oppression. The Declaration has indeed a wider reference also, because the ethical issues raised by psychiatric medicine—including questions of involuntary certification, detention and treatment of patients who, because of the nature of their malady, are incapable of giving informed consent—are acute even in countries where the basic human liberties are legally established. Indeed, it is sensitivity to these liberties which makes the ethics so sharp.

MEDICINE IN DEVELOPING COUNTRIES

All these initiatives arose in the developed countries, where the new medical science, and the new technologies based upon it, also arose. The developing countries are by no means forgotten. The expansion of Western medicine accompanied the combined imperialist, economic and missionary expansions of the nineteenth and early twentieth centuries. In some regions it replaced traditional practices; in others it coexists with them. In some countries attempts have been made to adapt Western organization of medicine and health care to local conditions and needs; in others, isolated centres of expensive high technology care stand out of widespread rural and urban deprivation. The mutation in medical science and practice has been slow, therefore, in the developing countries, for economic reasons and many others. Ethical concern shows itself in two directions in particular. One is to insist, so far as possible, that innovative or experimental procedures, like the trial of new medicines, vaccines or methods of contraception or of abortion, be conducted in poorer countries under the same ethical controls as are required in the richer and more developed—and the record of pharmaceutical promotion is by no means blameless in this matter.

The WHO/CIOMS guidelines specify the duty of close ethical cooperation with the host country, and the duty of training its health workers to work independently of expatriate control. The second ethical imperative is to insist that medicine has no frontiers: that advances pioneered in the developed countries be put at the service of those who need them in countries where medical services are still grossly inadequate, underfunded, understaffed. The contrast between the petty done and the undone vast is a grave moral issue. These twin duties are implicit in the WMA Recommendations Concerning Medical Care in Rural Areas, adopted in Helsinki in 1964 and amended at the Venice Assembly in 1983. The lack of provision for children whose expectancy of life and health is blighted by malnutrition and endemic disease is of particular concern; so is the need to assure that medical technology, and the organization of health care, are appropriate to the regions in which they operate, rather than modelled slavishly on exported experience.[14,15]

The aggressive marketing of breast milk substitutes and artificial babyfoods in these countries caused a setback, rather than an advance, in infant health. Not only did infants fed on substitutes lose the benefit of maternal immunities gained by suckling, but also the mixing of powders with water from infected supplies brought its own toll of disease and death. An *International Code of Marketing of Breast Food Substitutes* issued by the WHO from Geneva in 1981 was intended to abate the mischief. It aimed to encourage breast feeding, as in the best interest of the child and as an aid to the spacing of children. It advocated the control of marketing and advertising so as to reduce seductive or misleading pressures to change to artificial feeding unnecessarily. Positively it encouraged teaching in the right preparation and use of substitutes when they were necessary as a normal part of health care and education. Ironically, in the industrialized countries, where the choice between natural and artificial feeding is dictated more by fashion than by physical constraint, the return to the breast is now encouraged.

THE DISCIPLINE OF WORDS

Ethics should discipline words as it disciplines practice. The men of religion, philosophy and law have always been implicated with medicine. The doctors have sometimes found their presence obtrusive. Hippocrates contended for the liberation of medicine from superstition: epilepsy, 'the sacred disease', must have a natural cause, he argued, if only it could be found. Both he and Galen after him resisted the determination of pseudophilosophers and sophists to shackle science and medicine to their verbal systems. Theologians and philosophers, and men of other disciplines, participate in ethical discussions today; but there are dangers.

One danger lies in creating a new institution out of 'medical ethics', with its own specialists, 'medical ethicists', selfconscious, schematic, assertive, inadequately rooted in experience and practice, and usurping to itself a moral authority properly vested in others. The profession of theology or of moral philosophy in matters medical is ancillary—the office of a handmaid: it may not usurp the duties or the judgment proper to the profession of medicine. The relationship between them is most fruitful when practitioners invite these specialists, in small numbers, into the medical context where first of all they must learn, discourse, and think. Speculation is vain unless rooted in the realities of practice. 'Ethical' judgments are valueless unless they relate to those realities and can be implemented by those charged with the responsibility of decision. The practitioners themselves are the relevant moral agents: they are authorized by the community to take clinical decisions and to act on them, though that authority is now under challenge. Moralists are not so authorized; they can and ought to do no more than help to clarify the process of decision. They should strengthen and support the authorized moral agents of society, not undermine them. And when philosophers argue among themselves, in their domestic seminars and journals, divorced from the discipline of practice, they are the less useful to practitioners—however high their philosophical expertise, and however much they may advance thereby their own logical skills.

Lawyers, similarly, can dominate medical ethics to its detriment. Medical law is a necessity in a world in which justice has to be done. But the entry of the law, whether in civil or in criminal proceedings, only marks the breakdown of the ethical relationship which is primarily one of trust, voluntarily and mutually given. Medical ethics and practice now in the USA, and to a lesser but growing extent in Britain, are threatened with litigiousness.

Both invasions, the philosophical and the litigious, are encouraged by the artificial inflation of the rhetoric of 'rights'. That rights are sometimes genuinely in issue no reflective observer would deny. But 'rights' are now too frequently invented to clothe every fashionable aspiration or desire with legitimacy, with entitlement. They are invented, also, as though they were the only means of furthering good causes or of protecting the vulnerable. There is no need for this. We can express many of our moral obligations in the language of duties, without inventing rights. Animals, for instance, have no rights, in any strict use of the word; yet manifestly they have claims upon us and we have duties towards them because we know that they can suffer as we suffer; and laws exist to oblige us to treat them accordingly. The early embryo and the fetus have no rights, as the law understands rights: legal personality is not attributed until a child is born alive. Yet we have duties towards them, to protect them in their presumption in favour of life, and to take all positive steps to assure their wellbeing in the womb; and these duties the law will uphold. Confusion has swept into neonatal paediatric care from the assertion and uncertain acceptance of 'parental rights' even to deciding the destiny of the handicapped, whether they should live or die. Parents have *duties* towards their children. One duty is to assure in medical treatment that the best interest of the child is served or at least not threatened. Consultation with clinicians is entailed in the duty, as consultation with parents is entailed in the clinician's duty. But the only strictly relevant right of parents is to legal protection in the fulfilment of the duty.

Similar confusion arises from inflated talk about 'informed consent', even 'fully informed consent'. The doctrine as formulated in the US Court of Appeal in *Canterbury* v *Spence* (1972) is reported to have brought confusion and detriment to the theory and practice of law and medicine alike in some of the United States. The English House of Lords, in a judgment in *Sidaway* v *Bethlem Royal Hospital*, 22 February 1985, while affirming that a surgeon was under a duty to disclose to a patient any substantial risk involving grave adverse consequences inherent in the surgery or other treatment he was proposing, confirmed that the doctrine of informed consent, as enunciated in the *Canterbury* judgment, had no place in English Law.[16] It is for the patient to decide whether or not to consent to the treatment proposed for him by his doctor. But granted the limits to the possibility of non-medical persons being fully informed on medical matters, the real and effective basis of consent is not information but trust.[17]

Words matter. Respect for words, and discipline in their use, as discussed by Campbell in the next chapter, are essential for the proper expression of the next stage in the contemporary evolution of medical ethics. This is the education of patients, and of civil society, in their co-relative duties, their own obligations in relation to medicine and health care. The inflation of concepts by an undisciplined use of words creates false expectations, frustration and conflict. Ethics implies mutual obligations, a relationship of trust to which both parties covenant or commit themselves. A one-sided treatment of medical ethics, concentrating on the duties of doctors alone, leaves that ethics lame.

REFERENCES

1. Duncan, A. S., Dunstan, G. R., Welbourn, R. B. *Dictionary of Medical Ethics*. London: Darton, Longman and Todd; New York: Crossroad. Second edition, 1981: XXVIII.
2. The major codes are printed under *Declarations* in the *Dictionary of Medical Ethics*.[1] Periodical revisions are published by the World Medical Association.
3. Nicholson, R. H. (ed). *Medical Research with Children: Ethics, Law and Practice*. Oxford: Oxford University Press, 1986.

4. *Proposed International Guidelines for Biomedical Research Involving Human Subjects*. Geneva: WHO and CIOMS, 1982.
5. *Responsibility in the Use of Personal Information for Research: Principles and Guide to Practice*. London: Medical Research Council, 1985.
6. *Guidelines on the Practice of Ethics Committees in Medical Research*. London: Royal College of Physicians, 1984.
7. *The Confidentiality of Medical Records. The Principles and Practice of Protection in a Research-Dependent Environment*. EUR 9471 EN. Brussels and Luxembourg: Commission of the European Communities, 1984.
8. Iglesias, T. *In vitro* fertilisation: the major issues. *J Med Ethics* 1984; **10**: 32–37. (modified by Mahoney J. *Bioethics and Belief*. London: Sheed and Ward, 1984).
9. Dunstan, G. R. The moral status of the human embryo: a tradition recalled. *J Med Ethics* 1984: **10**: 38–44.
10. Edwards, R. G. The current clinical and ethical situation of human conception *in vitro*. The Galton Lecture 1982. In Carter CO (ed). *Developments in Human Reproduction and their Eugenic and Ethical Consequences*. London: Academic Press, 1983.
11. Council for Science and Society. *Human Procreation: Ethical Aspects of the New Techniques*. The Report of a Working Party. Oxford: Oxford University Press, 1984.
12. *Report of the Committee of Enquiry into Human Fertilisation and Embryology*. Cmnd 9314. London: Her Majesty's Stationery Office, 1984.
13. Saunders, Cicely M. (ed). *The Management of Terminal Illness*. Second edition. London: Edward Arnold, 1985. (See also articles on Hospice, Pain Control, Terminal Care in the *Dictionary of Medical Ethics*.[1])
14. Waterston, T. Appropriate technology: care of the newborn: a plea for closer monitoring of practice in under-developed countries. *Br Med J* 1984; **289**: 1229.
15. D'Arcy, R. F. Essential medicine in the third world. *Br Med J* 1984; **289**: 982.
16. Law Report. London: *The Times*, 22 February 1985.
17. Dunstan, G. R., Sellers, Mary J. *Consent in Medicine: Convergence and Divergence in Tradition*. Oxford: Oxford University Press, for King Edward's Hospital Fund for London, 1983.

Ethical Dilemmas in Health Promotion
Edited by S. Doxiadis

CHAPTER 2

Mere Words? Problems of Definition in Medical Ethics

ALASTAIR V. CAMPBELL

SUMMARY

'Words . . . slip, slide, perish, decay with imprecision, will not stay in place will not stay still.' T. S. Eliot.[1]

Clarity is required in the field of medical ethics in order to establish the definition of the subject area, the identification of an appropriate method of study and agreed usage for the central terms of discussion. Philosophical analysis can aid in this task, but it must be supplemented by substantive contributions from many other disciplines. In the specific area of the ethics of preventive medicine an interdisciplinary approach is required to tackle the following issues: the tension between personal freedom and the common good; permissible degrees of intervention in preventive medicine; the nature of the autonomy which constitutes human health and wellbeing.

INTRODUCTION

It often appears that in the discipline of medical ethics there is a fundamental *indiscipline*, a failure to use terms in a clear and consistent manner. To descend from the sublime words of T. S. Eliot to the more ridiculous argument of Humpty Dumpty in Lewis Carrol's *Alice Through the Looking Glass*—'When I use a word, it means exactly what I want it to mean—neither more or less'—this often seems the case with 'medical ethics'. Clearly such idiosyncrasy in the use of words renders any reasoned discussion of the issues of concern in modern health care quite impossible. It is necessary to find some common language which will allow people from different disciplines, and with different moral viewpoints, to communicate with one another. But where is such a language to be found? In this chapter I shall explore the contribution which might be made by philosophical analysis to such an endeavour. I shall consider three different areas of unclarity—the definition of the subject matter; the definition of the method; and the definition of the central terms which are used. No attempt will be made to enter into a full discussion of any of the specific issues arising in preventive health care, since these are dealt with in other chapters. Rather a general approach will be suggested, one which may help improve aspects of the discussion, but which is not intended to promote philosophy in any imperialistic sense. Philosophy, it will be argued, has a service function to perform and within medical ethics as a whole, but it is also of limited usefulness and must be complemented by the language and methods of other disciplines. This is especially true in the sphere of public health, since the issues raised are exceedingly complex and cannot be discussed adequately without recourse to political theory and sociological theory to set the ethical questions in an adequate context.

DEFINITION OF SUBJECT MATTER

The first problem which must be dealt with is the ambiguity of the term 'medical ethics'. Since this problem is dealt with at greater length by Dunstan and Karhausen in Chapters 1 and 3 of this volume, I need deal with it relatively briefly here. The difficulties are created partly by the many meanings given to the word 'ethics' and partly by the unresolved issues of whether *medical* ethics is a province specifically or exclusively belonging to the medical profession.

We may attempt to resolve the first difficulty by drawing a distinction, albeit a purely conventional and artificial one, between 'ethics' and 'morals'.[2] Ethics is to be regarded as the critical reflection upon morals. Thus it is not to be confused with the codes of behaviour subscribed to by the medical profession, nor is it to be confused with the opinions or beliefs of individuals or groups about what constitutes right conduct or good decision-making. Ethics uses codes, beliefs, opinions, decisions, guidelines as the raw material for its analysis, seeking norms by which to judge the coherence and the adequacy of these constituents of the morals of groups and individuals. Thus ethics is a critical discipline, at one stage removed from the day-to-day choices of morality. But (ideally at least) the critical reflection which it offers should improve the quality of the decisions made. Special note should be taken of the place of religion in the origin and maintenance of moral beliefs and moral behaviour. In a pluralistic society it is necessary to find a shared set of moral convictions which are not conditioned by one particular religious belief. Thus medical ethics must be self-sustaining, not dependent upon the Christian or any other religious faith. On the other hand, the powerful influence of religion in creating a sense of communal identity and responsibility and in helping individuals to follow their moral commitments cannot be ignored.

It will be obvious from this definition of ethics that medical ethics should not be regarded as the special preserve of the medical profession. While it is true that many of the decisions which affect the moral quality of medicine are decisions which doctors alone can make, even within this reserved professional area doctors themselves may not be the best critics of the decisions which are taken. As a special interest group it is inevitably difficult for them to distinguish between what is of benefit to the profession (and confirming of the special viewpoint of their discipline) and what is of benefit to the individual or the society as a whole. Moreover, many of the most urgent questions arising from the practice of medicines are ones which go far beyond specifically medical expertise. This is clearly the case in preventive medicine, perhaps more than in any other field, because of the socio-political character of the issues of debate and because any decision-making must take into account broad sociological and psychological factors related to attitudinal change in individuals and in whole societies. In this field medical expertise, which relates to the understanding and elimination of disease and disability, is only one of many disciplines which are required. There is no reason to suppose that medical specialists will be the best qualified to judge which preventive interventions (designed to improve the health status of a group or designed to raise the general standard of health within society) are morally justifiable interventions.

In view of these difficulties, would it be advisable to discard the term 'medical ethics' in favour of a less misleading description? The most commonly used alternative is 'bio-ethics'. Yet this carries with it all the problems of a neologism. Since its meaning is not self-evident, it has to be defined for those not familiar with its use. Why then not stay with the more familiar medical ethics, supplying the necessary corrective to those associations which make it appear non-critical and professionally biased? Moreover, the prefix 'bio', which is intended to refer to the 'life sciences' tends instead to create a misleading impression that *biological* issues are paramount in the discipline. This may indeed have been a danger in the United States where the term is most commonly employed, since there has been a tendency to avoid the socio-political dimensions of health care and to focus on the scientific and the individualistic relationship between doctor and patient. An interesting example, illustrating this tendency, is described in a recent paper[3] suggesting guidelines for the teaching of medical ethics in the USA, compiled by a group of experts on the subject. The group could not reach unanimous agreement that 'knowledge of issues in the equitable distribution of health care' should be in the basic curriculum. But the real difficulty with the term medical ethics remains that, in modern Western societies at least, the medical profession holds a position of special authority and power in all activities associated with the art of medical care, even although many other professional groups, many non-professional groups and patients themselves may have equally important parts to play. This suggests that a broader and professionally more neutral term should be employed. For this reason the phrase 'health care ethics', or (more pedantically but also more accurately) 'the analysis of moral issues in health care' is perhaps preferable. Such phrases imply that there *are* issues requiring critical analysis and the question of who is competent to debate them is not foreclosed.

DEFINITION OF METHOD

We turn next to the method which should be used in order to develop a critical ethics which will improve the quality of discussion of the many moral issues which arise in preventive health care. Here we must scrutinize the term 'critical'. It refers to the ability to make judgments (Gk: *krisis*). The judge in the law court, the referee in a sporting contest, the art, drama or literary critic, each is recognized as a competent person to judge within that sphere what is correct or incorrect, sanctioned or not sanctioned, of greater or of lesser quality. But who are the expert judges of *moral* quality? This is a question as ancient as the Socratic dialogues and as elusive of a simple answer, then as now. It is easier to see the forces which destroy moral integrity than to describe how it is to be promoted, for, it is evident that as soon as one group in society sets itself up as the moral arbiter, two attitudes corrosive of morality develop—prejudice and hypocrisy. It is as though human beings are incapable of carrying the weight of authority for judging the morality of their fellow humans without that weight itself distorting their viewpoint. Each time a group sets itself up as those who possess the necessary *krisis* in morality—whether that be a priestly caste, a political elite or a body of professional experts—there comes a narrowing of the perception of the good to the limited vision of a fallible few. The dangers of hypocrisy and of moral elitism are aspects of human nature which Christianity, based on the teachings of Jesus against Phariseeism, has been quick to point out. Paradoxically however, it is often those who hold strong Christian beliefs who are the first to fall into these errors. History is full of examples of attempts by the Church to exercise moral control on the society as a whole.

It seems, then, that the salvation of a truly critical ethics is that no-one should be regarded as a 'moral expert'. This is presumably what Socrates meant when he said that he was wise only in that he knew that he knew nothing. But how, then, are judgments to be made? How is it possible to make any progress in ethics, if no-one is an expert? In answer to this, we must consider carefully what it might mean to develop a method in ethics which is genuinely interdisciplinary in character. For, it could be that by locating the 'expertise' in the dialogue between disciplines, we can avoid the damage of one group claiming expertise. It could be, on the other hand, that we merely compound confusion!

In order to consider how ethics can be interdisciplinary we must examine briefly the distinction between fact and value. It is sometimes naively supposed that subject areas can be divided between the sciences concerned chiefly with the establishment of facts and the humanities concerned chiefly with questions of value. In such a division the place of the 'human sciences'—psychology, sociology, politics—is problematical. Are they hard sciences dealing with well-established facts? Or are they inevitably value-laden and so at the soft end of knowledge, closer to aesthetics or even theology? Increasingly, such categorizations are being regarded as inappropriate because of the demise of the belief in 'value-free' science. At the basis of every scientific investigation, it is now recognized, there are certain assumptions about the nature of reality which themselves cannot be proved and which may indeed be totally set aside by a 'revolution' in science of the kind brought about by Einstein. To say that science is closer to reality because its theories are productive of technological innovation is, of course, to provide an answer of a kind to the question 'are scientific theories true'? But such an answer does not avoid value judgment. It is a commitment to a naive form of pragmatism, asserting that that which is true is that which 'works'. The effect of this approach in medicine is all too evident.

Thus the debate about values should always be a debate *across* disciplines, with all participants recognizing that they start from certain assumptions which are rarely questioned within their own discipline, but which can fruitfully be questioned when outsiders ask about their theories and their conclusions. It has become clear in recent years that medical ethics has awakened from its dogmatic slumber precisely through this process, since medical practitioners and medical scientists have become increasingly willing to share their clinical decision-making and their theoretical advances with a wider group. A clear example of this would be the lively debate which has developed around new advances in reproductive medicine, such as *in vitro* fertilization and experimentation on the human embryo. There is a growing realization that the perceptions of pure science alone are not sufficient to guide society about what should and what should not happen in this field. The same point should surely hold for the ethics of preventive medicine. Here is a field which involves epidemiologists, educationalists, sociologists, political theorists, medical practitioners in numerous specialities, philosophers and theologians. Each group has something to say about what would bring greater benefit in terms of an improved level of health in society. But each has preconceptions about the nature of health and about what contributes to human progress. Only when the implicit values are subjected to mutual scrutiny can there be some hope that a moral absolutism—whether based on a narrow scientism or on an unchallenged philosophical or religious dogma—will be forced to yield to an approach which seeks to be open to the whole range of available facts and to see the complexity of the value judgments involved. The need to defend one's assertions to practitioners in another discipline is a powerful antidote to a simplistic view of the moral problems which confront us in implementing policies in preventive medicine.

In this context the discipline of philosophy can be seen to have a specific function to play—but it is far from a master role! On the contrary, it is to be viewed primarily as a service function, as a means of improving the quality of the communication between disciplines, without itself providing any very specific contribution to the answers which must be sought. For, unlike all the other disciplines involved, philosophy has virtually nothing to contribute by way of content. Rather, it is concerned with the logical structure of arguments, with the consistency with which terms are employed, with the clarity or otherwise of their definition, and with the coherence (or lack of it) between the starting points and the conclusions of arguments. Thus philosophy is primarily (though not exclusively) analytical, and as a result it is a parasite upon the other disciplines. If no one made any assertions about fact and value then the philosopher would have nothing to analyse! But it must be added that this account of philosophy is a little too bare. For the legacy of philosophy includes a long history of metaphysical speculation which provides a rich source of ethical theories of various types. Thus the philosopher is also in a position to recognize theoretical stances of various types, which keep reappearing in various forms throughout history when people make assertions about moral principles and moral values. Obvious examples of this are the mutually contradictory assertions that all morality is based on the pursuit of happiness and that the moral law requires obedience whatever one's desires. Such a historical perspective provides the philosopher with a set of categories by which the theoretical assumptions of contemporary debates can be more quickly recognized. Most arguments in morality have a déjà-vu quality about them—little seems to have changed since Socrates encountered his sophistical adversaries in the dialogues constructed by Plato! But this knowledge of ethical theories does not put the philosopher in a superior position in the debate about moral priorities. If this debate is to be more than a mere sport, a game with words, then choices must be made. When it comes to drawing conclusions the philosopher is as vulnerable to error as anyone else. For moral choice entails commitment to some set of values in a situation which is by definition one of uncertainty and dilemma. If everything were clear and self-evident, what would be the need of debate?

DEFINITION OF CENTRAL TERMS

We come now to the application of this approach to method in health care ethics to the specific area of preventive medicine. I shall avoid a detailed exposition of any one issue, since all these to which I shall refer are dealt with at greater length elsewhere in this volume. My task is merely to indicate why certain issues are important, if the morality of prevention of ill-health is to be adequately discussed.

The challenging aspect of this area of medicine is that it renders obsolete the emphasis in codes of medical ethics on the relationship between *individual* patient and *individual* practitioner—for example, the first clause of the Geneva Convention Code: 'The health of my patient will be my first consideration'.

Admittedly, it is possible to focus attention on preventive measures which remain within the individual doctor–patient relationship, such as therapy which prevents recurrence, advice to patients on healthy life-styles, and so on. But by far the most effective and most controversial aspect of preventive medicine is that which seeks to influence the health of whole populations through measures ranging from education and advertising on the media, to mass prophylactic measures (immunization, screening) and legislative controls on behaviour (seat belts, control of marketing of alcohol and tobacco). It is in the public health aspect of preventive medicine that the controversial ethical issues arise. Indeed the problem is that this is largely unknown territory for ethics as a whole. Traditionally ethics has dealt with examples of culpable action (murder, theft, lying), whose effects on human wellbeing are little in doubt. But preventive medicine is concerned with probable outcomes, whose precise effects are often hard to predict, either in terms of the balance of positive and negative effects or in terms of the numbers of people likely to be affected, beneficially or adversely. This makes the choices much more difficult to assess morally, every option being coloured as much by political ideology as by commitment to more personal moral values. Nevertheless, despite these complexities, the issues must be identified and dealt with as best we can with the intellectual tools available to us.

The first set of issues concerns the relationship between the individual and the state and focusses upon the rights and the obligations of citizens. Within this context the key terms at issue are 'the common good' and 'personal freedom'. The second (closely related) set of issues concerns the relationship between the providers and the receivers of services and focusses upon the tension between autonomy and paternalism. Within this context the key terms at issue are 'education', 'intervention' and 'health'. I shall consider each of these sets briefly in turn, from the perspective of an interdisciplinary approach to health care ethics which uses philosophical analysis and ethical categorization as a heuristic device for aiding decision-making.

The first set calls for no less than an exploration of the character of democracy—a highly complex and contentious area in political theory. But the debate cannot remain in the realm of theory. It also requires the input of historians of medicine and of epidemiologists to illustrate the major impact upon the health of individuals brought about by general social change and by health legislation. This in turn requires a careful analysis of arguments about freedom. Is the individual entitled to a freedom which damages the health prospects of others? Is freedom to be regarded as a personal possession or as a quality of life, in terms of opportunity for wellbeing, which is spread evenly across the population? Is freedom to be defined negatively (non-interference with one's wishes) or positively (enhancement of human potential)? Again, if rights entail obligations, what obligations does the individual citizen have toward the society which grants him or her certain rights? Finally, does the government of a democratic state have a mandate to raise the general state of health and wellbeing in the society by legislative measures which restrict the freedom of groups—for example, marketers of products—if their activities, though not illegal, can be shown to be health destructive? When this set of issues is more carefully examined, it becomes obvious that few if any of these questions have simple yes or no answers. Rather each resolves itself into a question of *degree*—how much personal freedom as opposed to legislative control? and so on. Thus virtually all countries have *some* health and safety legislation, but controversy arises about how restrictive of market forces such legislation should be—for example, in relation to processed food or to pharmaceuticals of dubious value. It is because such questions are tied up with relativities, not with absolutes, that the interrelationship of disciplines is so important. The social scientist and the epidemiologist can speak with some authority about social trends, predictable risks and so on. But these projections need the critique which comes from health practitioners, who see the practical outcomes of unhealthy social conditions—and both groups need help from political and social philosophers in discussing what would be morally acceptable within the framework of democratic process. No single discipline could conceivably provide the necessary expertise across this range of topics.

Lurking within this first set of issues is a major problem in political philosophy—how is 'democracy' to be defined? The term has become a catchword for wildly divergent political views, ranging from the people's democracies of the Eastern Bloc, with a single party as the voice of the people, through the complex array of parties in coalition in some Western European countries, to the two-party system largely characteristic of Britain and the USA. Behind this diversity there is a single crucial issue, the nature of political representation. Who speaks for the people? And how is the welfare of the state to be enhanced, if the will of the majority opposes that which appears beneficial to those better informed of the facts? Clearly the 'despotism of the majority' (as J. S. Mill put it) has great dangers, but equally dangerous is the accumulation of power to influence people's lives by a sub-group, whether they be political activists, the commercially powerful or those who can claim the status of 'expert'. It seems that social benefit is best served by a form of democracy which has sufficient checks and balances built into it to prevent any one interest becoming inappropriately powerful. But it is not yet clear what the details of such a system would be in order to ensure a democratic approach to preventive measures in health care. At present, this aspect of medicine is slow to gain wide acceptance and it has problems in gaining real political force, when commercial interests are ranged against it. We are still a long distance from a real emphasis on prevention becoming a political priority within parliamentary democracies, and far less in the world as a whole where few compromises between competing political systems are ever achieved. Thus preparation for war remains a priority and the soluble problems of worldwide disease and poverty are spasmodically dealt with, if at all.

The need for interdisciplinary discussion is equally, if not more strongly, evident in the second set of issues. What are the justifiable methods of influencing people's behaviour and life-style apart from those which can be given legislative force? We may hesitate to use the heavy control of law in some areas where personal freedom appears paramount—but may we then attempt to use persuasion, and, if so, what type of persuasion is morally acceptable? The dilemma in this topic area is at its greatest when we realize that there is ambiguity in a quite central aspect of this whole question—how health is to be defined. If we were secure in our definition of health, then it might be easier to describe the potential role of health educationalists or health promoters. But in fact health is itself so tied up with individual expectation and attitude that it defies simple definition. Thus, for example, the end result of some 'health education' about heart disease or about diet could be simply to make people more anxious and more obsessed about their bodily state, thus *reducing* their health prospects. A further problem stems from the centrality of 'autonomy'—a capacity for self-direction and a sense of dignity—to a state of health. For how can methods of persuasion, modelled on advertising techniques, promote autonomy if they work covertly upon people, rather than enabling them to take independent decisions about their life-styles? It may appear that the persuasive aspects of preventive medicine are doomed to be either ineffective (because too careful not to interfere with the autonomy of others) or counter-productive (because effective by methods which remove the autonomy of others). To resolve such a dilemma it is essential to examine carefully the nature of the relationship entailed in genuine change as opposed to manipulation. In this context a number of theoretical perspectives have a part to play—studies of the character of relationships in the health and welfare professions, educationalist theory (particularly within the sphere of adult education), media studies, studies of religious evangelism, and theoretical perspectives on health, especially in its social and psychomatic dimensions. This kind of interdisciplinary work, if focussed on specific questions—such as change in dietary habits, use of leisure, attitudes to family life—could lead to some provisional answers to the major health issue in modern post-industrial societies. How can we help people become active participants in their own good health and in the improvement of the health of the communities in which they live? Such an outcome can be brought about only when the agency of individuals is safeguarded and enhanced by the activities of those involved in preventive medicine.

CONCLUSIONS

In this brief survey of the nature of ethical discussion in preventive medicine I have sought to go beyond 'mere words' to the identification of the principal issues in the field, to a suggestion about an appropriate method for discussing them in a critical and creative way, and to a general description of the subject area.

My conclusions may be summarized as follows:

1. The aim of ethical reflection on health care issues is to provide the basis for decision-making based on as comprehensive and critical a survey as possible of the subject area.
2. No single profession or academic discipline can claim an expertise in this field. Consequently discussion must be interprofessional and interdisciplinary.
3. Philosophical method has a specific service function to perform in the discussion, consisting of a clarification of the concepts employed and a categorization of the types of argument.
4. The main moral issues arising within the field of preventive medicine can be grouped into two sets: (i) the rights and obligations of citizens, contained in the apparent tension between personal freedom and the common good; (ii) the relationship between the initiators of preventative measures and their target groups, specifically as this affects that component of health described as autonomy.
5. Most of the issues resolve themselves into questions of degrees of intervention or non-intervention rather than into simple yes or no answers. For this reason there can be no substitute for the complex and inevitably provisional suggestions for action which emerge from interdisciplinary debate.

REFERENCES

1. Eliot, T. S. *Four Quartets*. London: Faber and Faber, 1974.
2. Campbell, A. V. *Moral Dilemmas in Medicine*. Third edition. Edinburgh and London: Churchill Livingstone, 1984: Chapter 1.
3. Culver, C. M., Clouser, K. D., Gert, B. *et al*. Basic curricular goals in medical ethics. *N Engl J Med* 1985; **312**: 253–56.

Ethical Dilemmas in Health Promotion
Edited by S. Doxiadis

CHAPTER 3

From Ethics to Medical Ethics

LUCIEN KARHAUSEN

SUMMARY

Ethics is the philosophical discipline primarily concerned with the evaluation and justification of norms and standards of personal and interpersonal behaviour. Justification is a rational procedure and ethical principles should be consistent and capable of universal application. The language of ethics is primarily prescriptive while the language of science is descriptive. This fundamental distinction shows why ethics cannot be deduced from science nor medical ethics from medical science (naturalistic fallacy). The history of ethical doctrines is long and complex but there are two main currents—deontological and utilitarian. The link between these two approaches and the two basic disciplines concerned with people's health—medical practice and public health—will be shown. Finally, the relationship and the tension between ethical principles ('ethics') and the general public's ethical beliefs ('morals') will be discussed.

INTRODUCTION: HUME'S LOGICAL GAP

A theory of ethics is essential to all of us if only in distinguishing for us the difference between what we do and what we ought to do. But any consideration of an ethics of a science, such as medicine, immediately faces difficulty and tension because the language of ethics is primarily prescriptive while the language of science is descriptive.

This can be illustrated by the following quotation from David Hume which has become known as his 'guillotine'[1] and which is often summarized by stating that one can never derive an ought from an is:

> 'In every system of morality, which I have hitherto met with, I have always remark'd, that the author proceeds for some time in the ordinary way of reasoning, and established the being of a God, or makes observations concerning human

> affairs, when of a sudden I am surprised to find, that instead of the usual copulations of propositions, is, and is not, I meet with no proposition that is not connected with an ought, or an ought not. This change is imperceptible; but is, however, of the last consequence. For this ought, or ought not, expresses some new relation or affirmation, it is necessary that it should be observed and explained, and at the same time that a reason should be given, for what seems altogether inconceivable, how this new relation can be a deduction from others, which are entirely different from it. But as authors do not commonly use this precaution, I shall presume to recommend it to the readers; and am persuaded, that this small attention would subvert all the vulgar system of morality' (*Treatise of Human Nature*).

Hume's seminal remark has been interpreted as trying to point out the fundamental distinction between saying on the one hand that an end is being pursued or a moral principle is being actually followed and on the other hand that the given end ought to be pursued or that the moral principle ought to be applied. Psychology or sociology, being scientific disciplines, may describe or explain how individuals or groups of people do behave and what their beliefs are concerning their own behaviour, while ethics says how they ought to behave.

Hume's remark got support from modern logic: the two modes of speaking are deductively independent. The indicative mode, illustrated by scientific discourse which describes and explains, is of a different nature from the prescriptive mode of ethics or of politics. Moreover a prescriptive statement, for instance an ethical claim, can never be logically derived from an indicative statement unless the latter explicitly or implicitly contains some prescriptive element.[2,3,4]

That cigarette smoking causes lung cancer can be supported by facts, in the present case by epidemiological evidence. But one cannot provide evidence of this kind to support the value statement 'Cigarette smoking is bad'. We can observe cigarette smoking and we can observe cancers but we cannot observe badness. Thus, the following reasoning is illogical: (1) Cigarette smoking causes cancer; (2) Therefore cigarette smoking ought to be curbed. However, the addition of a further premiss would make it valid. (0) We ought to eliminate causes of cancer. Now the conclusion (2) which contains an 'ought' follows logically from premisses (0) and (1) which also contain one 'ought'.

The main philosophical point to be drawn from this is that ethical matters and ethical decisions cannot be deduced from mere scientific facts and that no additional scientific research is going to solve ethical questions, and in particular, medical ethical questions. This of course does not mean that medical facts are irrelevant to medical ethical issues—it is simply that scientific discourse is of a descriptive nature while ethical discourse is of a normative or prescriptive nature.

FROM VALUES TO ETHICAL VALUES

Ethics in fact is a philosophical discipline mainly concerned with the critical evaluation and justification of norms of personal and interpersonal conduct.

Moral agents are responsible agents and it is assumed that they are able to form plans, give reasons and make rational choices which are most likely to lead to their goals.

Practical reasoning[5] consists in finding means to the end. But good practical reasoning will not guarantee that the action will be a moral one. There are good and bad reasons for action and there are good and bad goals. Therefore a rational theory of action and of decision is merely the beginning of a theory of morality. We have to agree about what are good reasons and what are good goals. This shows where values and normative claims enter the picture. Moreover rational practical reasoning supposes that our goals or our ends are internally consistent so that there will be a continuing need to integrate and coordinate our ends. Will such procedures for practical reasoning be sufficient to guarantee moral behaviour? It does not seem so. The *Highway Code* satisfies those requirements of practical reasoning but it does not thus become part of moral laws.

The question then is: what more is needed? Is there any specifity in moral behaviour which distinguishes it from other forms of rational behaviour? Does morality have a point? Some authors have provided a positive answer to this question,[6] but however we try to resolve this issue, one major element remains necessary in order to transform good behaviour into moral behaviour.

If ethical principles were merely accepted ways of behaving, differing social practices related to different cultural patterns would represent different moral standards. Ethics would become a mere chapter of sociology and morality a sum of local cultural conventions relative to some populations at a given moment of time and history. This would also collapse the logical gap of David Hume. But ethical relativism is untenable since it actually refutes itself. Ethical relativism claims that there should be fundamental differences in the moral standards of different communities or of different cultural groups. This is a normative claim which applies to all societies all of the time and which demands that normative claims do not apply to various societies all of the time!

This leads us to one of the central and most fundamental conditions of moral claims which is their universality. Moral principles should be universal or at least universalizable. Kant[7] wrote 'So act that the maxim of your will could always hold at the same time as a principle establishing universal laws'. For instance no act of lying is right. If everyone lied continually deception would be a universal feature and nobody would believe a promise whether it was a true or a false promise. The liar would find himself in the inconsistent situation of willing to deceive and willing a universal law prohibiting the deception.

Talent, abilities, social roles and a particular background are certainly relevant to the specification of what actions are to be performed and what moral principles are being followed. What Kant meant was that a given action is a moral action for a person if, and only if, the same action is morally permissible for any person in the same situation. Of course Kant's principle is often going to fail or to be misapplied but this is irrelevant to its cardinal function in moral reasoning.

Human action can have instrumental or intrinsic value.[8] Judged according to their instrumental value actions may be desirable or undesirable as a means to further ends. On the other hand, if they are judged according to their intrinsic value their desirability or undesirability is an end in itself and of itself.

Utilitarian Ethics

The first ethical approach, which is usually described as utilitarian, claims that whatever is conducive to the maximization of pleasure and happiness in society is good—that is, the greatest happiness of the greatest number. This, simply expressed, is the ethics of consequence.

The general spirit of this theory concerns social welfare, and of course health, but also freedom, democracy and justice. The value of the consequences of rules or actions determines the moral nature of ethical rules and principles and of ethical actions. Ethical concepts can be translated into quantitative measurable terms such as health, pain, pleasure, justice . . .

Moreover these welfare dimensions can also be measured in terms of their extent—that is, the number of people affected by them.

This first approach, favoured by Jeremy Bentham[9] and John Stuart Mill,[10] judges human actions by evaluating their consequences, especially their quantifiable aspects. Generally speaking, it assumes that actions or policies are right or wrong according to the extent to which they contribute to promote the human welfare (or the welfare of all sentient beings) of all those concerned. Values are to be agreed upon and they are extrinsic or instrumental: we may like to promote the greatest happiness, the greatest pleasure, the lesser suffering or the greatest health for the greatest number. I should behave in such a way that my action maximizes the total amount of pleasures and minimizes the total amount of pain of those persons affected by the action (counting each person as one and no person as more than one).

Deontological Ethics

The second approach considers that acts or rules are good or bad regardless of consequences and is called deontological, from the Greek *deon*, meaning obligation or necessity, the ethics of duty. A given behaviour is ethically right not because it leads to desirable consequences but merely because it is obligatory, because it is an irreducible duty. This is often expressed by saying that people ought to behave according to the dictates of their conscience which refers to their moral sense.

This second approach, that of Immanuel Kant[7] or of the Torah, considers some actions and practices to be intrinsically valuable, and stems from a concept of moral duty and from a concern to treat people as ends rather than solely as means. I should behave in a certain way for the sole and sufficient reason that it is my duty.

THE ETHICS OF AESCULAPIUS AND THE ETHICS OF HYGEIA

These two doctrines of utilitarian and of deontological ethics have their counterparts in health care. Let us first look at the use we make of the concept of effectiveness in medicine and in health care. The effectiveness of antihypertensive preventive therapy was clearly established in a randomized controlled trial conducted by the Veteran's Administration, some of the results of which are summarized in Table 1.

Table 1 Relative effectiveness of antihypertensive preventive therapy.

Baseline mean diastolic pressure (mmHg)	Percentage with non-fatal events		Percentage attributable population effectiveness per 100	Relative effectiveness
	Control (*a*)	Treated (*b*)		
90–104	25.0	16.3	35	1.1
105–114	31.8	8.0	75	1.3
115–129	35.7	2.7	92	1.5

In terms of absence of non-fatal events, relative effectiveness of antihypertension therapy versus placebo is $100\text{-}b/100\text{-}a$—for example, $(100\text{-}16.3)/(100\text{-}25) = 1.1$. Percentage attributable effectiveness is expressed by $100(a-b)/a$. Relative effectiveness is expressed as the ratio of the proportion without events and under combination therapy (thiazide, reserpine, hydralazine) to the proportion without events with placebo. Population attributable effectiveness of the treatment is the difference between percentages of incidence of events in placebo and treated groups divided by percentage incidence in placebo group. Now the relative measurement is mostly relevant to clinical care and to individual patients.

Clinicians who wonder how effective hypertensive drug therapy is, tend to think in terms of relative effectiveness. In the present study relative effectiveness is low in mild diastolic hypertension but it increases with the severity of the hypertension.

On the other hand, population attributable effectiveness taking account of the chosen end points is very significant and it allows the public health officer to expect a substantial benefit if one assumes that the proportion of hypertensive persons in the general population is about 12 per cent. Instead of being expressed in terms of personal risk, the expected benefit is now expressed in terms of number of lives improved or of avoidable non-fatal cardiovascular accidents.

The relative measurement describes effectiveness from the viewpoint of the patient and of the clinician. The attributable dimension shows by what amount, in terms of number of persons and of morbid events, a given health problem will be improved in the population.

The clinician who weighs the benefits of chemotherapy in solid tumours or the best surgical approach to gliomas of the central nervous system thinks in terms of relative effectiveness for the individual patient. A public health administrator goes for what he considers less trifling questions, such as whether aspirin ought to be widely distributed to those who survived a first myocardial infarction, and of course his main concern relates to attributable effectiveness for his health population.

There are interventions which have a high attributable effectiveness but a low relative effectiveness—for instance, the administration of aspirin in the post-myocardial infarction syndrome. Such interventions may be very attractive for public health policy but somewhat less so for a clinician in direct relationship with his individual patient.

Another illustration concerns the concept of risk. Risk estimates may be expressed in two ways reflecting two distinct medical philosophies (Table 2).

Table 2 Comparison of relative risks from lung cancer and from coronary heart disease for heavy smokers and non-smokers.

	Lung cancer	Coronary heart disease
Annual death rates (per 100 000 persons)		
(a) Heavy smokers	166	599
(b) Non-smokers	7	422
Relative risk to heavy smokers	166/7 = 23.7	599/422 = 1.4
Risk attributable to heavy smoking (per 100 000 persons per year)	166–7 = 159	599–422 = 177

Relative risk relates the disease rate among smokers to that in non-smokers. Non-smokers become ill as a result of exposure to factors other than smoking. Relative risk, therefore, gives us an estimate of the causal relationship which links smoking with cancer of the lung—the higher the ratio the stronger the association and the stronger the case in favour of a causal relationship.

Coronary heart disease, on the other hand, presents a very different picture with a much lower relative risk suggesting other causal factors.

In brief, it appears that population attributable indices are expressed in terms of additive units (usually sick persons) such as number of deaths, number of persons improved, or number of morbid events. This is precisely why they are particularly useful for the decision-maker. There are numerous such indices: effectiveness, safety, harm or risk. Population attributable indices are connected with universalizable utilitarianism which is the main moral foundation of most preventive and public health policies.

On the other hand the relative indices express the probability of some sort of desirable or undesirable event and their use therefore relies on deontological bases.

It is generally acknowledged that relative indices such as relative risk are a better index of causal relationship than attributable indices. Once it is known that an observed relationship is a causal one, then the attributable risk gives a better idea of the quantitative social impact of a given programme.[11] More generally, relative indices are of more interest to clinicians. When deciding how to treat their patients, doctors are looking more or less explicitly for relative effectiveness while a community health physician is more interested in attributable effectiveness. Occupational physicians need indices of relative safety or risk of the worker's environment while occupational health managers need attributable indices. The risk of occupational accidents may be quite small as far as the individual worker is concerned but may pose a significant risk in industries at large. Relative indices are therefore highly relevant for medical practice, doctors and patients—that is, within a situation ruled by an ethics of duty and respect for person.[12]

Screening procedures attempt to identify presumptive unrecognized diseases or defects by the use of high sensitivity methods: this actually means that screening procedures do accept a high percentage of false positives. It is therefore better, in utilitarian terms, for a screening procedure to identify healthy individuals as sick than to pass some of the sick ones as healthy.

The situation is much more complex in a deontological-clinical approach where it may be important either not to treat a healthy subject for a disease he does not have, or else where it is important not to miss any case of a disease which is 100 per cent curable. Diagnostic tests may need either to be highly specific or highly sensitive.[13] Diagnostic methods, as opposed to screening methods, are essentially patient-centred. There are many examples of the two traditions of health care, the Hippocratic one, based on the doctor-patient relationship and the collective one with its stress on prevention and optimization and distributive justice.

Public health is essentially utilitarian. Resource allocation has a strong tendency to favour those health care issues which represent a heavy burden in terms of suffering, morbidity and mortality and rare diseases are more likely to be neglected. The case of the so-called orphan drugs[14] is an interesting illustration of this point. Orphan drugs are those drugs whose development is not cost-effective so that industry needs 'some reimbursement for technical development and other major costs'. This is only one aspect of the difficult problems related to an equitable distribution of medical research and health care resources.[15] Discussions on these issues often underline the point that a fair distribution of resources will complement utilitarian principles with some sort of principle of equity.

Ethical concepts are inevitably omnipresent and pervasive in medicine, and medicine and public health can be seen as chimaeras trying to link or to weave in two families of concepts separated by an unbridgeable logical gap. If ethical statements are neither true nor false but right or wrong, or justified or unjustified, what happens when they are combined with scientific statements which are true or false? If the 'is' and the 'ought' are closely interwoven how can we talk about medical ethics? This is a difficult philosophical problem and here I propose simply to make a few clarifying points. Danto[16] has shown that it is not regarded as a failure in a discipline such as medicine or among its practitioners, if one cannot answer external questions about the discipline itself; it is enough if doctors can answer internal questions which are properly medical to be successful practitioners. Internal questions in medicine are questions about aetiology, treatment, prevention, health management. Medical ethics raises external questions: what is just health care? is prevention a form of paternalism? is killing a malformed newborn baby immoral?

In other words, ethical issues being deeply ingrained in the fabric of medicine and of its language cannot be analysed within medicine or within its language. They can only be discussed and analysed from an outside point of view, from what might be called a 'metamedical' position. It is impossible to analyse a practice within that same practice without removing the critical discourse outside that practice. The latter manoeuvre recreates the logical gap between medical language (or medical practice) and the language within which it is analysed and discussed which is essentially a philosophical one. As soon as we talk about medical ethics, medicine becomes a moated castle.

THE DISCIPLINARY IDENTITY OF MEDICAL ETHICS

These considerations lead inevitably to the conclusion that medical ethics is no more a medical discipline than a legal or theological one. What we have to face up to and accept in any practical consideration of medical ethics is that ethical philosophy is not going to provide unequivocal answers to moral questions. We cannot avoid the issues but we must look further and deeper than scientific fact to resolve them. And we must be prepared for difficulty and discomfort.

Subsequent chapters contain numerous descriptions of existing practices which are being taken as points of departure for ethical discussion. Moreover sociologists' talk about medical ethics is significant and relevant. If this is so what are the consequences and where do we stand in view of what was said about Hume's guillotine?[17] Did not Hume warn us about the dangers of moving, and thus of inferring, from descriptive to prescriptive discourse?

The morality of a particular social group is a plain social phenomenon and there are objective and concrete criteria for determining its rules. Morality is often seen as unwritten law and the same can be said for moral beliefs. But this type of moral discourse seems to lack an essential ingredient since it merely describes facts and does not interfere with individual behaviour.

Ethics on the other hand does not come in the indicative but in the imperative mode: 'this ought to be done' stems from a point of view which is both in and of society. Much of the current literature on medical ethics moves back and forth from indicative (external and descriptive) language to the imperative mode (internal and normative or prescriptive). Of this we must beware, or at least aware since it introduces the risk of confusion. But it also has the merit of displacing the emphasis from a mere matter of moral rules towards the essential striving of morals: trying to bridge the gap between ethics and conduct. Discussions about medical ethics tend to be not so much about what ought to be done or about what is being done as about the relation between them.

The changing content of moral judgments is the result of a process of mutual adjustment of principles and social judgments going back and forth from theory to practice, from ethical theory to social mores, until a coherent view is reached which takes account of and is consistent with personal and general current moral sentiment. In this book we are concerned with various aspects of the relationship between ethics and practice in preventive medicine, and, as throughout the history of western morals, this relationship remains one of a tension between what there is and what there ought to be.

REFERENCES

1. Hume, D. *An Enquiry concerning Human Understanding*. Library of Liberal Arts. Indianapolis: Bobbs-Merrill, 1960.
2. Moore, G. E. *Principia Ethica*. Cambridge: Cambridge University Press, 1903.
3. Hudson, W. D. *The Is-Ought-Question*. London: MacMillan, 1969.
4. Putnam, H. *Fact and Value in Reason, Truth and History*. Cambridge: Cambridge University Press, 1981.
5. Raz, J. *Practical Reasoning and Norms*. London: Hutchinson, 1975.
6. Foot, P. Moral arguments. *Mind* 1958; 502–513.
7. Kant, I. *The Groundwork of the Metaphysics of Morals*. (Translated by Paton, H. J.) New York: Harper and Row, 1975.
8. Aristotle: *Nichomachean Ethics*.
9. Bentham, J. *An Introduction to the Principles of Morals and Legislation*. 1838.
10. Mill, J. S. *Utilitarianism*. Library of Liberal Arts. Indianapolis: Bobbs-Merrill, 1970.
11. MacMahon, B. and Pugh, T. F. *Epidemiology, Principles and Methods*. Boston: Little Brown and Company, 1970.
12. Roberts, C. J. *Epidemiology for Clinicians*. London: Pitman Medical, 1977.
13. Galen, R. S. and Beyond, S. R. *Beyond Normality*. New York: John Wiley and Sons, 1975.
14. Editorial: Therapeutic Orphans. *Lancet* 1985; **2**: 702–703.
15. Scheinberg, I. Investigating diseases no one's got. *N Engl J Med* 1985; **309**: 918–919.
16. Danto, A. *What Philosophy is*. New York: Harper and Row, 1968.
17. Brinton, C. *A History of Western Morals*. New York: Harcourt and Brace, 1959.

Ethical Dilemmas in Health Promotion
Edited by S. Doxiadis

CHAPTER 4

Origin of Modern Public Health and Preventive Medicine

A. H. M. KERKHOFF

SUMMARY

The history of public health and preventive medicine is not simple to analyse and less simple to understand. It is more closely related perhaps than curative medicine to changing cultures and the processes of civilization. The nineteenth century saw the foundation of modern public health based on utilitarian principles. In this chapter the background to this is examined with a basis in the humoral theory of Ancient Greece and the idea of the influence of physical and biological environment on health and the much later realization that social environment might also be important. The foundations of administrative structures essential to the successful introduction of a system of public health are also discussed. The role of the state is an area which has continued to present dilemmas for preventive medicine and this is shown to have evolved very differently in various European countries. The historical overview suggests that nineteenth century utilitarianism can still provide powerful guidance for collective preventive medicine today.

INTRODUCTION

Even a superficial glance at today's health care systems shows a strong tension, not only between moral and non-moral motives but also between the various ethical concepts. The friction between distributive and aggregative theories in particular provokes entirely new problems. An extensive ethical approach, therefore, seems indispensable.[1] For this purpose the ethicist needs in the first place to define the moral domain—he has to consider the actions against the background of the available possibilities. It must be clear, however, that in defining this moral domain, consulting with medical historians will not be his first choice of action. The only material the latter can offer consists of what the past may contribute to a better understanding of today's situation.

The task which the medical historian takes on is far from simple. He cannot limit himself to summarizing preventive actions as such. Collective preventive medicine presumes the intervention of government. This means that he must look at these actions as one part of public health care, in other words, of the total package of governmental activities in relation to public health. The history of public health care is not simple to analyse and less simple to understand. The German medical historian Julius Pagel observed that this history is closely related to the culture and processes of civilization, more so even that is the case with the history of curative medicine.[2] This difficulty is enhanced by the fact that the history of public health has a capricious course, with the differences of culture and even of country so large that a general survey would result in a major textbook. In this chapter, therefore, I intend to limit myself—if not in geographical terms, then at least in chronological terms. Since the nineteenth century saw the foundation of modern public health, the developments of that period can enlighten us best with respect to the present situation.[3]

The history of public health during the nineteenth century, however, has been amply discussed by many others and it would be difficult to add much to the existing knowledge. Even the question of why public health developed so vigorously during the nineteenth century seems to have been answered satisfactorily. Brockington, for instance, states that a climate of opinion emerged which was more favourable to public health. This in turn was based 'more upon enlightened self-interest than on visionary dedication'. 'The development of a social conscience', he adds, 'followed when disease or squalor were seen to endanger the lives and health of rich and poor alike . . . ' This, according to the author, resulted in a change of governmental attitude with regard to public health care: 'the absence of recognition by authority of any precise obligation to develop public health services' disappeared.[4]

These opinions are no longer new. Nevertheless they maintain stimuli for the medical historian, and possibly for the ethicist as well. They imply that public health did not develop by virtue of new medical knowledge but rather because of changes in attitude with respect to the duties and responsibilities of governments. It seems worthwhile, therefore, to analyse the thoughts of Brockington, who certainly does not stand alone in his opinion, once again and to test them where possible.

How can one test these ideas? One opening might be offered by an ethical principle: ought implies can. This means that we should first investigate if the ingredients necessary for an effective public health system existed before the time in which men like Sir Edwin Chadwick did their magnificent work. If they did, then it would be an indication that changes in social attitude rather than medical developments were responsible for the rapid rise of public health care in the nineteenth century.

What, therefore, is required for the administration of adequate public health? Superficially, the answer to this question appears to be clear—effective medical methods such as Jenner's vaccination against smallpox. On closer analysis, however, the answer is more complicated. Preventive measures are often important against diseases for which no cure has yet been found, usually because of insufficient insight into the particular pathophysiology. There must also be at least a feasible medical theory which enables a systematic search for effective measures.

A second consideration in this context is that we usually think first of medical measures when talking about the prevention of disease. But, as McKeown has described so strikingly, many important measures in the field of public health were not of a purely medical nature. Improvements in nutrition, housing and working conditions are good examples of non-medical measures which have had an enormous effect on public health.[5] So we cannot limit ourselves to measures and examples from medicine, but are compelled to extend our field of interest to the social domain.

Knowledge of effective methods, or feasible theories at least, is thus a necessary but not sufficient prerequisite for an adequate public health system. The measure must also be capable of being brought into effect and this means that the government must have an adequate administrative apparatus.

Finally, we must not forget the question of motives. Was it true that governments, before the nineteenth century, did not consider public health care as part of their responsibility?

UNDERSTANDING THE NATURE OF DISEASE

As mentioned before, effective preventive measures are often the result of deliberate and systematic research. This presumes a workable medical theory, explaining a maximum of phenomena with a minimum of suppositions. Such theories have coexisted in the past in many forms. The supranaturalistic opinions are very ancient. These theories are not founded in the laws of nature, but arise from a world of thought not limited by confirming experience—the world of deities, ghosts and demons. The iatro-theological concept of disease played a paramount role in preventive health care models. In essence this theory is governed by the concept that disease is caused by disobedience to the Master.[6] This concept is mentioned in biblical works as well as in Homer's *Iliad*, in which an angry Apollo launches his pestiferous arrows onto the Greeks in order to punish them for the rape of a priest's daughter. The iatro-theological theory has never disappeared entirely. Even today traces remain as, for example, recently when a high-ranking clergyman stated on Dutch television that the threat of an AIDS epidemic ought to be seen as a punishment of God.

In the present context, however, the naturalistic theories are of greater importance. They consist of certain conceptions about the physical nature of man in relation to the complex of structures and forces in his environment. A theory of special interest in this context is miasmatism, the concept which guided Chadwick when founding the sanitary movement. In order to understand this theory in greater depth we have to go back to Ancient Greece where humoral pathology emerged. Broadly speaking, this theory held that the human body is a reflection of the surrounding cosmos, a microcosm in the middle of a macrocosm. The elements of the macrocosm (water, air, earth and fire) are found in the human body as humors: mucus, blood, black and yellow bile. According to this theory, the humors should be present in their correct proportions and relationships. Illness was seen as a disturbance of the harmonious balance of the humors.[7] This disturbance, according to the *Corpus Hippocraticum*, could be caused by an unhealthy way of life. While this was responsible for individual diseases, the cause of epidemics was sought in climate, seasons, water, and the nature of the soil. The influence of the air was thought to be of even greater significance as it was the most common element. It could become polluted (miasma is derived from *μιαίνω*: to pollute) and thus affect large numbers of people at the same time. It was on the basis of this theory that, according to Thucydides, the Athenians lighted high fires when their city was tried by pestilence.

It is clear that humoral pathology was very effective in disease prevention. It taught the importance of a good diet and a sensible way of life in general. It also explained why living in cold and humid places was unwholesome and why swamps had to be avoided. It should not surprise us then, that humoral lore, and miasmatism as its derivative, were of great importance until far into the nineteenth century—the members of the sanitary movement applied miasmatism with considerable success.

THOUGHTS ON THE SOCIAL GENESIS OF DISEASE

In the previous section we saw that long before the nineteenth century theories emerged which were quite practical in the context of preventive medicine. They concerned the influence of the physical and biological environment on man and his health. The idea that interaction with the social environment might also be significant for disease and health is of a much later date. Not until the era of the Enlightenment did this idea become defined. One of the greatest men of that time was Jean Jacques Rousseau (1712–1778). Although he was not a physician, he may be considered among the founding fathers of public health. His versatile mind, which cannot be classified within one discipline, became famous by answering a question posed in 1749 by the Academy of Dyon: 'if the reestablishment of arts and sciences had contributed to improvement and elevation of morality?', with a forceful no. In his reply Rousseau doubted the value of culture—whereas most of his contemporaries lauded its blessings. The arts and sciences, according to Rousseau, are not milestones of progress but, by contrast, commemorate decay. Could we not dispense with lawyers if, by virtue of cultural refinement, injustice had not been introduced into life? Would we need physicians if the complex of culture, rules, regulations and conventions did not cause disease? In his *Discours sur l'origine et les fondements de l'inégalité parmi les hommes* (1754) Rousseau goes into the question of disease in greater detail distinguishing between those of natural origin, such as diseases of old age, and those of non-natural origin, such as those caused by social conditions.

> 'With respect to disease; I shall not recount the empty and false allegations which are brought against medicine by most healthy men. But I do pose the question if adequate studies have been made, based on which one may conclude that the average lifespan is shorter in countries where the art of medicine has been neglected, in comparison to those countries where medicine is practised at a high level of refinement. How could we do so where we are known to inflict more diseases upon ourselves than may be cured by medicine? The most incongruent ways of life, complete idleness of the one as compared to excessive activity of the other, the ease with which our senses are provoked and with which these provocations are being satisfied, the extravagant food of the rich, giving rise to heartburn and causing indigestion as opposed to the inadequate nutrition of the poor, causing them to glut when given a chance, the night-revelling, various extravagances, the unlimited explosions of passion, the fatigue, the mental exhaustion, the sorrow and the endless griefs, gnawing constantly at men of all classes, all this guarantees in a fatal way that most of our ailments are self-inflicted and could have been avoidable had we adhered to the simple, regulated, and solitary way of life which nature prescribes'.[8]

These were Rousseau's basic ideas about pathogenesis. He considered moral corruption to be the root of all evil. How could this situation be improved? His criticisms on culture have to be seen against the background of his thoughts on man in his natural state.[9] Nevertheless the philosopher saw that merely taking off the shrouds of culture did not offer a solution. Man must regain his natural freedom in spite of the denaturalizing influence of culture and civilization. It must be possible to develop a governmental policy according to which natural freedom is brought into harmony with the powers necessary to guarantee political order. For this purpose the '*contrat social*' forms the instrument of choice—each member of society submits himself to the supreme command of the community as a whole, with all of his rights and all of his powers. This community is a political one, for, like Plato, Rousseau saw the political community as the surest means of effecting freedom—not from the state but from the disease-producing society. 'It is of the essence of society', he wrote in a letter to Mirabeau 'to breed incessant war among its members; and the only way of combating this war is to find a form of government that will set the law above them all'.[10]

A major part of the value of Rousseau's contribution to public health must be attributed to his thesis that disease is an attribute of social circumstances. He made clear that disease is not only the result of a disturbance in the balance of humors but also the result of the disturbance of the harmonic balance between social forces. Rousseau's influence has been immense. Not only did he inspire politicians to far-reaching reforms, but he also put his stamp on the line of thinking of philosophers as well as some physicians. Among them is Johann Peter Frank, who is considered by many as the father of the '*Medizinische Polizei*'.[11] Focusing on the German scene once more, the thoughts of men like Neumann and Virchow on social misery and disease can be associated directly with Rousseau's line of thinking. [12]

Thus it seems clear that a usable theory about the social genesis of disease was present in Chadwick's time although not greatly before it. The question of whether these thoughts were known to the great reformer is not difficult to answer. It can be extracted from his earliest writings. It is less easy to discover to what extent his ideas were derived directly from the French 'philosophes'. In his writings Chadwick indicates that he based his opinion on his own observations. True as this may be (as a student he focussed his attention on newspaper articles about the London slums), there is no doubt that his thinking was influenced at least indirectly by the ideas of Jeremy Bentham.[13] Before going into this matter in further detail, we must first look at the origins of the infrastructure necessary to administer preventive medicine.

FOUNDATIONS OF ADMINISTRATION

The presence of practical theories are thus an absolute prerequisite for measures in the field of public health and preventive medicine. In order to enable the government to carry out the actions an administrative apparatus is necessary as well. To identify the foundations of administration we must go back to the beginnings of the post-medieval era. In the Middle Ages implementation of public health measures had been reasonably simple. The lines of command were short, and the links between the various members and layers of the small municipal communities were clear and tight. This changed when larger modern states emerged. With the increase in scale, the process of government became more complex.

The nobility had an important influence on the emergence of national states. They tried, often without shunning the use of great violence, to carry on their medieval policies, albeit on a larger scale. Political justification for their endeavours to subject entire nations was found in Absolutism, which held that a sovereign has the complete power over country and subjects on grounds of a divine right. In order to be able to exert his power down to the lowest level, the sovereign had to use the intervention of civil servants, but this did not solve all his problems. Centralization of power implies the search for a suitable form of bureaucratic machinery, and a theory and practice of administration. Thus a new discipline emerged; the name of which is best translated out of the original language as 'policing sciences' (*Polizei-Wissenschafte*).

Among the protagonists of this new science was Melchior von Osse (1506–1556) who was commissioned by the Elector of Saxonia to write a monograph about this subject. A second important personality was Georg Obrecht (1547–1612) who wrote a similar work half a century later, in which he elaborated on the value of proper registration of population growth by means of recording births, marriages and deaths. Although his work was a significant step forward it was Veit Ludwig von Seckendorff (1626–1692) who defined the absolutist attitude of the state with respect to public health care.[14] The absolutist sovereign had to promote the health of his subjects in order to increase his powers. To maintain and increase his powers a large military organization was also of prime importance. For this purpose large numbers of healthy subjects were necessary as well as sufficient finances. The latter could only be achieved by increasing production for which a healthy labour force was a prerequisite. The fields as well as the means mentioned by Seckendorff represent a complete health programme which would not be out of place in many states today. His programme consisted of the training and supervision of midwives, the care of orphans, and the appointment of physicians to combat infectious diseases. He also described in detail the quality control of nutrients and water, as well as the cleaning of streets and canals.

ROLE OF THE STATE

There were many authors from this period who dealt with public health against the background of medical police. This was not only the case in absolutist Germany and France, but also in England, where Mercantilism induced a similar health policy.[15] Becker was one of the first authors in whose work we recognize the spirit of Enlightenment. In his *Politische Diskurs, von den eigentlichen Ursachen dess Auff- und Abnehmens der Städt, Länder und Republicken* (1669) he states that a government should be subject to the people.[16] This line of Enlightenment thinking has been of the greatest significance for the development of public health service. Part of it we have already seen in Rousseau's ideas on the sociogenesis of diseases. Its influence, however, extends much further. The rational approach of the Enlightened philosophers led to a better insight into the anatomy and physiology of the state which in turn benefited the structure of the medical administration. More importantly, the Enlightenment cast new light upon the aims and functions of public health service and especially upon the role which government had to fulfil.

Among the principles of the Enlightenment was the conviction that all men are free and equal. It was in this context that many philosophers directed their attention to the political structures of society. They rejected Absolutism. Where the teachings of Absolutism included that the state was personified by the sovereign, the Enlightenment reasoned that people were free and therefore sovereign themselves. As a consequence the sovereign must look after the interests of his subjects above all. This point of view meant an important change in the way of thinking about public health and its aims. Furthermore, the Enlightenment no longer accepted public health care as a means of enlarging the power of the sovereign. Instead it introduced the idea that promoting health should serve the interest of the individual citizen, which in turn would serve the general interest.

This thought was implemented in different ways in the various European countries. France needed a Revolution to realize the concept of freedom, equality and fraternity, and its medical implications. In Germany the Enlightened thoughts of the philosophers were hybridized with Frank's concept of medical police and substantiated in what Frank himself called 'System einer vollständigen medizinischen Polizei'. While his ideas were adopted by the Hapsburg Emperor Joseph II, the developments in Great Britain were entirely different. Here the teachings of Adam Smith (1723–1790) were of great influence. He stated that an invisible hand would steer the general interest as long as everybody looked after his own welfare. In accordance with the individualistic spirit of that time he rejected any governmental interference: in contrast to Frank he felt that the latter could only inhibit and disturb social and economic progress.

UTILITARIANISM AS A BASIS FOR MODERN PUBLIC HEALTH CARE

Thus the knowledge which proved to be necessary in the nineteenth century to form the basis for public health service, was already available by the end of the eighteenth century. There was in miasmatism, a usable medical theory, there was a clear insight into the sociogenesis of disease and there was a sufficient amount of knowledge on the workings of a governmental machine. Last but not least, understanding of the relations between man and society had deepened and the possible role of the government had been studied in various ways. But though all necessary prerequisites had thus been satisfied, almost another half century was to pass before modern public health care was established. One may wonder why government did not act at an earlier stage—50 years is a long time in terms of the social abuse as well as the countless diseases in England in those days. We do not need to look far to answer this question—libertarianism reigned supreme, meaning that the state abstained from intervention as much as possible. Therefore, we must conclude that Brockington was right in the sense that new medical inventions did not give rise to public health care. Changes in attitude about the tasks and responsibilities of governments did. Why did these attitudes change? The answer to this question is perhaps most effectively provided by a scrutiny of Jeremy Bentham's line of thinking—the ideas of Chadwick and many other advocates of the sanitary movement did indeed originate from the circle of this lawyer-philosopher.

Bentham's philosophical thoughts do not occupy much space in the handbooks. His greatest merits—according to recent publications of the physician-philosopher

Ten Have—lie not so much in the originality of his philosophy as in the fact that he initiated, partly through his students, important political and social reforms.[13] At a young age he already contemplated reforming penal law, an ideal which had possessed many Enlightened thinkers. It was this way of thinking which determined Bentham's philosophy. He fervently studied the work of the French 'philosophes' and corresponded with men like d'Alembert, Mirabeau and Voltaire. Closely related to his striving for a better penal system were Bentham's views on the good and evil of acting, both by individuals as well as by governments. Bentham soon became a staunch supporter of the utilitarian principle, described in chapter 3 by Karhausen, which taught that good or evil are determined by the greatest possible happiness in the largest number of people. With the 'greatest happiness principle' Bentham meant: 'that principle which approves or disapproves of every action whatsoever, according to the tendency which it appears to have to augment or diminish the happiness of the party whose interest is in question: or, what is the same thing in other words, to promote or to oppose that happiness'.

This thought was not entirely new. Indeed, the writings of the French Enlightened philosopher Adrian Helvetius, induced Bentham 'to regard the principle of utility as an oracle, which if properly consulted, would afford the only true solution that could be given to every question of right and wrong'.

Bentham did not limit the application of the utilitarian principle to the immediate domain of penal law. It also became a leading principle in his thoughts on society and on the place and task of the state. In his thinking, society is a fictitious body, consisting of individual members. This largely determines the relation of interests between individual and society: the interest of a society is the sum of the interests of its individual members. Individual interest comes first in this system: it results from what is also known as psychological egoism—man is always in pursuit of his own happiness.

This principle of self-preference is embraced wholeheartedly by Bentham—he even states that man would cease to exist as soon as individual interest no longer came first. Nevertheless the philosopher is of the opinion that the ethical norm for action should be different, and that man should pursue general happiness or better still, the greatest happiness of the greatest number.

This obviously presents a difficult problem—how can utilitarianism be the norm, if egotism is the practice? The answer which Bentham gives to this question is that of an Enlightened Philosopher: one should presume that the interests of people are naturally in harmony. This means that the greatest happiness of the largest numbers can be achieved if everybody pursues his own greatest happiness. In turn, it also means that man is serving his own purpose when in pursuit of the greatest happiness for the largest number.

To propagate these thoughts, Bentham attached great value to the legislators. The central place of the greatest happiness for the greatest number, in Bentham's philosophy, determines the aims of the law as well as the responsibilities of the state and the legislator. Bentham did not regard the state as a super-entity with its own aims, but as the democratic product of the people, meant to enable them to realize their wants and relationships as well as possible. The ideal form is representative democracy—only this can realize the greatest happiness formula. It should not—contrary to what libertarianism taught—abstain from interference, but take action. This means that it maintains security, supplies means, and, last but not least, promotes equality. Next to fighting poverty, the promotion of public health is the important feature. The means, mentioned by Bentham in this context, are not new. The state must protect the people against poor medical care, must guard over water and air as potent sources of disease, and moreover, must—how could it be different in the eyes of this Enlightened rationalist?—supply information about healthy ways of life.

The directives given by Bentham in this context could have been taken directly from the *Corpus Hippocraticum* or from the works of Galen: among other things they pertained to proper and balanced diet and no excess of any kind. Furthermore, they included good ventilation and temperature regulation, and, something which was quite often lacking in those days, 'no unhealthy occupation, no excessive labour prescribed or so much as permitted'. This classic advice takes us back to where we began. It was not new medical concepts which gave rise to public health care in nineteenth century England. The utilitarian thoughts as propagated by Bentham and his followers were new indeed. They gave leverage to the new developments and thus set them in motion. One might argue that this all passes over the great significance of the effect of the diseases themselves, especially of cholera. Virchow called cholera the ally of hygienists since it stirred governments to actions and awakened social conscience. Indisputably the role of disease has been large. It must be considered, however, in the proper context. One should bear in mind that Bentham introduced with utilitarianism a philosophy already present in pre-revolutionary France long before the cholera epidemics took place.

It is true also that Bentham can hardly have been influenced by the incidence of the disease. The first epidemic took place when he was almost 80 years of age. It appears more practical to assume therefore that the dreaded cholera may have contributed to a faster acceptance in larger circles of the thoughts of Bentham and his students. Moreover, cholera should be regarded as part of a larger complex of changes, brought about by the industrial revolution. The new industrial resumption of society implied more generally that people were more dependent on each other than had been the case in agricultural and pre-industrial societies.

CONCLUDING REMARKS

This diversion into history seems to corroborate the idea that the principal stimulus to the development of modern public health care was a philosophical one. This certainly is not a fresh idea. Nevertheless, it seemed worthwhile to put forward this view once again. We must continue to realize that public health in the nineteenth century was based on utilitarian principles. The fact that, in the meantime, medical science has made considerable progress—even more than in any period before—does not diminish the importance of this fact. After all, the many new discoveries do affect curative, rather than preventive medicine. As to the prevention of cancer, coronary heart disease and chronic degenerative disease, medical knowledge has not yet improved so much. In that respect little has been altered. As Campbell has shown,[1] even the fact that the health care problems of today can no longer be solved by applying exclusively utilitarian principles, does not remove their value: most of the problems he refers to concern the curative part of medicine. In the field of collective preventive medicine utilitarianism still can serve as a feasible and powerful guide.

REFERENCES

1. Campbell, A. V. *Moral Dilemmas in Medicine*. Edinburgh and London: Churchill Livingstone, 1972.
2. Pagel, J. L. *Einführung in die Geschichte der Medizin in 25 Akademische Vorlesungen*. Berlin: S. Karger, 1915: 552.
3. Chave, S. P. W. The origins and development of public health. **In**: Holland, W. W., Detels, R. and Knox, G. (eds). *Oxford Textbook of Public Health*. Oxford, New York, Toronto: Oxford University Press, 1984; **1**: 3–20.
4. Brockington, C. F. The History of Public Health. **In**: Hobson, W. (ed). *The Theory and Practice of Public Health*. London: Oxford University Press, 1971: 1–7.
5. McKeown, T. *The Role of Medicine*. Oxford: Basil Blackwell, 1979.
6. Rothschuh, K. E. *Konzepte der Medizin in Vergangenheit und Gegenwart*. Stuttgart: Hippocrates Verlag, 1978: 21–46.
7. Schöner, E. Das Viererschema in der Antiken Humoralpathologie. *Sudhoffs Arch* 1964: **5**.
8. Guillemin, H. (ed). *Du Contrat Social*. Paris: Union Générale d'Editions, 1973: 306.
9. Beerling, R. F. *Het Cultuurprotest van Jean-Jacques Rousseau*. Studies over het thema pathos en nostalgie. Deventer: Van Loghum Slaterus, 1977: 56.
10. Nisbet, R. *The Social Philosophers*. New York: Washington Square Press, 1983: 45.
11. Lesky, E. Einleitung zu Johann Peter Franks Akademischer Rede vom Volkselend als Mutter der Krankheiten. (Paris, 1790). *Sudhoffs Klassiker der Medizin*; **34**. Leipzig: Barth, J. A., 1960: 7–29.
12. Jacob, W. Aus dem sozialmedizinischen Erbe Rudolf Virchows. Medizin als Wissenschaft vom Menschem, *Revue Internationale de l'Histoire des Sciences de la Medecine, de la Pharmacie et de la Technique* 1965; **52**: 218–240.
13. Ten Have, H. *Geneeskunde en Filosofie*. De invloed van Jeremy Bentham op het medishe denken en handelen. Lochem: De Tijdstroom, 1983: 180.
14. Rosen, G. Cameralism and the concept of medical police. *Bull Hist Med* 1953; **27**: 21–42.
15. Rosen, G. Economic and social policy in the development of public health. An essay in interpretation, *Fr Hist Med All Sci* 1953; **8**: 406–430.
16. Schwartz, F. W. Idee und Konzeption der Frühen territorial-staatlichen gesundheidspflege in Deutschland ('Medicinische Polizey') in der ärztlichen und staatswissenschaftlichen Fachliteratur des 16–18. Jahrhunderts. (Thesis). Frankfurt am Main, 1973: 92.

Ethical Dilemmas in Health Promotion
Edited by S. Doxiadis

CHAPTER 5

Why Prevent Disease?

ROGER BLANEY

SUMMARY

The ideas inherent in disease prevention strategies are of great antiquity but have become more complex in recent times, partly related to the changing pattern of disease. Various models have been created to explain the existence of disease and belief in such models may influence the type of preventive strategy being used. When the term 'prevention' is used in its broadest sense the distinction from treatment becomes much less clear. Just as in the clinical situation, however, public health interventions require justification. Many factors militate against prevention, some relate to what the public see as an imposition and others to questions of individual freedom.

INTRODUCTION

While the idea of prevention as generally welcomed may appear straightforward enough, it is necessary to discuss some of the underlying concepts in what has also been described as 'anticipatory medicine'. Although diseases, injuries and causes of death are unanimously considered as being undesirable it does not necessarily follow that every attempt to avert the occurrence of disease will be universally acceptable. What is meant by prevention requires to be considered and preventive strategies need to be justified. In this chapter my aim is to outline a reference framework against which ethical problems may be seen in the context of preventive ideas and philosophies.

DEVELOPMENT OF THE PREVENTIVE CONCEPT

The idea of maintaining health by prevention is of great antiquity. The Bible, the classic of ancient records concerning disease, places greater emphasis on the prevention of disease than on treatment, and the ancient Hebrews by amalgamating their own concepts of hygiene with those of the Egyptians, were the first to devise a code of hygiene.[1] From the concept of the sick individual as it first appeared in primitive civilization, 'hygiene' came to include consideration of the welfare of the group, first of the family, then of the nation, and then of the world at large—a true social concept.[2] The wholescale application of preventive measures to total populations had to wait for the development of appropriate political structures, however, and such changes in Europe along with discoveries about the environmental origins of disease (e.g. scurvy) preceded the monumental works of Johann Peter Frank (1745–1821), the 'Father of Public Hygiene', who tried to systematize the health knowledge of his day and showed how this might be applied through government action for the benefit of the people.[3] Despite the absence of a translation into English, Frank's influence was wide and long-lasting. In 1798, for example, Dr Andrew Duncan (1744–1828) wrote a memorial on State Medicine for the University of Edinburgh, Scotland explaining the principles of 'Medical Police',[4] and a paper read by Henry Maunsell (1806–1879) before the Royal College of Surgeons in Ireland in 1839 on the subject of 'Political Medicine' led to his being appointed in 1841 as Professor of Hygiene or Political Medicine in the same College, the first chair in this subject (now called Community Medicine) in Great Britain and Ireland.[5] In addition to these developments the coincidence of other factors underlined the importance of preventing disease. The dreadful epidemic of cholera that spread throughout Europe in the early 1830s created the urgent necessity of collecting vital statistics. In England, it was the analysis of these statistics by Chadwick, Snow, Farr and others which identified the disease as being caused by contaminated drinking water and the associated insanitary conditions of the crowded towns and cities. Helped by the rising tide of philanthropy the numerous preventive strands were brought together into the great Public Health Movements of the nineteenth century.

The very success in controlling, and in some cases eradicating, the major epidemic diseases has cast doubts paradoxically on contemporary possibilities for prevention. The greatest health problems in the Western World are now chronic non-contagious diseases, which appear to originate in the habits and behaviour of citizens themselves. The issues nowadays seem less clear-cut and many governments protest their reluctance to curb unnecessarily the freedom of individuals 'for their own good'. There has been a commensurate rise in the promotion of health education which aims at changing behaviour by giving information and by changing attitudes.

MODELS OF DISEASE CAUSATION

The theoretical principle underlying the possibility of primary prevention is the 'Causal Principle'—that is, that every event (in this case disease) in the universe depends for its occurrence on a definite set of conditions, necessary or sufficient.

To many the Causal Principle is a 'necessary truth' and not open to empirical disproof. Presumably such people would be more optimistic in the pursuit of aetiological factors.

Sets of shared ideas about causal mechanisms have been described as models or paradigms. Each model views the development of disease from its own standpoint. In earlier times people were more likely to believe that diseases were the result of attacks by evil forces in the form of spirits or demons and that the solution was to practise various rituals including sacrifice. The belief in one God saw the world as ruled by His Providence. The Bible recounts clearly how epidemics and plagues could be sent as an expression of the divine wrath of Jehovah. The Moral Model of disease emphasizes the role of Providence and prescribes fasting, prayer and moral practice as a method of deliverance. The Marxist Model employs the theory of dialectical materialism to explain disease processes. The Health Belief Model discussed later underlines the importance of individual health perceptions in determining risk-taking behaviour.

The advent of the bacteriological era introduced the Infectious Disease Model which emphasized the agent–host–environment interaction. Robert Koch (1843–1910) laid down 'postulates' for establishing the pathogenicity of a particular organism (agent) as a necessary condition for the disease in question: (1) the micro-organism must be observed in every case of the disease; (2) it must be isolated and grown in culture; (3) the pure culture must, when inoculated into a susceptible animal, reproduce the disease; (4) the micro-organism must be observed in, and recovered from, the experimentally diseased animal. It was soon realized that a pathogenic organism, although a necessary condition for the disease, was not in itself a sufficient condition, and that the state of the environment as well as susceptibility in the host were important additional factors in understanding infectious disease causation. It is the interaction between these three elements of the model which explains the origins and predicts the spread of communicable disease. It also points towards measures for prevention and control. The same model has been successfully applied to the understanding of accidents and trauma where the agent instead of being an organism becomes an 'undesirable transfer of energy'. This model, while placing trauma problems in their ecological setting, identifies the agent as 'an environmental entity whose action is necessary to produce the specific damage of interest and without which it cannot occur'.[6]

With chronic non-communicable diseases where there are prominent aetiological agents, such as tobacco or alcohol or other physical or chemical substances to be incriminated, the model may also fit reasonably well. For other chronic diseases, however, such as coronary artery disease and various cancers, the necessary causal conditions have not been discovered. In these the concept of agent is weakened and the host–environment factors may interact through a series of sufficient conditions. The science of epidemiology attempts to unravel the interacting causative factors and to decide whether each factor is independent, confounded, additive, synergistic or antagonistic. In coronary artery disease, for example, no predisposing factor has yet been identified as being necessary for the disease to occur. The term 'risk factor' is therefore used instead of 'cause' and no factor can be identified as equivalent with an 'agent'. Risk factors have not met the criteria laid down for a cause, such as (a) adequate strength of statistical association between the factor and the disease, (b) occurrence of the supposed cause to precede in time instances of the supposed effect, (c) 'production' of the disease in a controlled experiment, (d) consistency with existing knowledge.[7] It must be acknowledged that absolute proof is impossible and that it is unnecessary for prevention to know the actual mechanism of the causal relationship.

In theory the difficulty in identifying causal relationships between various factors and disease may lead some to reject the Causal Principle. The principle can never be disproved, because the discovery of more causes is taken as confirming it, but failure to find causes disturbs it not at all.[8]

STRATEGIES FOR DISEASE PREVENTION

Although it is useful to describe the problem in terms of necessary and sufficient conditions, prevention will be more directly related to causation as such. Being alive, for example, is a necessary condition of contracting tuberculosis, but it is not a cause. In devising prevention strategies priority is given to the identification of causal factors which are amenable to manipulation. A balanced view is required to decide whether a given factor is causal or not. It is suggested that intervention should be economic, acceptable, feasible, effective, efficient and carry negligible side-effects.

In order to clarify the issues involved, consider the case of a man-eating tiger attacking a village community. True primary or first level prevention would mean capturing or killing the animal and stopping permanently any further maulings or deaths. The swiftness of the intervention would also determine the final number of deaths prevented. However, neither the weapons nor the organization required are available to this small community. The alternative equivalent action would be to evacuate the village but the cost may seem too high. Not being able to eradicate the cause of their distress, a second level strategy would be to create protection. A fence, barrier or shield around the village, while not eliminating the cause, would afford protection but with significant restriction of movements and interference with the freedom of village life. The men of the community, however, are so tired out and taxed with the preoccupation of individual defence, shutters on windows, treating and transporting the wounded, that this crowds out any more strategic action. The people do their best but in the absence of leadership, organization and resources it is practically a case of everyone for himself. As individuals are powerless against the animal, the tiger continues to terrorize the village and claims many victims particularly the weakest. In this theoretical example the problem continues for years so that villagers accept that the proximity of this deadly animal is a part of their normal existence. A system of rules of behaviour grows up ('never go out alone at night'); there are early warning systems; and the villagers have become very skilled in the treatment of wounds.

In our own society as well there would appear to be an immediacy about everyday crisis intervention which would tend to divert attention from the essential humaneness of planned strategic action. The analogy could be used of the military leader who is so busy keeping the enemy at bay that he is unable to plan his campaign.

THE MEANING OF PREVENTION

To prevent means to take action in advance, to take measures before the untoward event occurs in order to stop it happening. Clark distinguishes between prevention in a narrow medical context when it means averting the development of a pathological state and the broader sense of limiting the progression of disease at any stage in its course.[9] Epidemiologically, prevention in its basic sense means to reduce or abolish the incidence of disease—that is, the rate at which new cases of the disease arise. The concept is modern because historically evil forces (including disease) were inevitable and human effort was directed towards avoidance or averting catastrophe. Therefore true first level prevention eliminates the origins of the disease itself, whereas prophylaxis, protection against disease, and disease avoidance are aimed at strengthening the resistance of the individual or group against disease onslaught.

It is common to describe prevention in terms of primary, secondary and sometimes tertiary forms. The distinction is that primary prevention is the approach aimed at reducing incidence of disease while secondary prevention aims to reduce prevalence by shortening the duration. Tertiary prevention is defined as aimed at reducing complications.[10] There are some difficulties about this classification. For example, although vaccination and immunization described as primary prevention may eventually reduce the incidence of disease in a population by limiting its spread, the best example being the eradication of smallpox, they nevertheless operate through protecting individuals rather than attacking the cause of disease. Similarly, seat-belts may protect the wearer against injury and death but do not affect the accident rate. And the problem is that many clinicians use the term secondary prevention to describe measures taken—for example, exercise, stopping smoking, diet—to reduce the chances of a further attack of a disease. Prevention is often contrasted with treatment but therapeutic intervention can have preventive aims—for example, 'to prevent death'.

The concepts involved might be better understood and categorized by considering four relevant aspects of prevention, the object, subject, methods and responsibility. The *object* of intervention may be to prevent disease, disability, death (premature or imminent), or a second attack of the same disease. The *subject* of preventive action may be the individual, a group or a total population. *Methods* may range from compulsory legislation (wearing of seat-belts, fluoridation), to clinical procedures such as physical examination or administration of a drug. *Responsibility* for preventive action may rest with an individual physician, the patient, healthy members of the population, with employers, with health services or with government. Strictly speaking, therefore, it is only by the objectives that we can decide that a measure is 'preventive'. In practice, however, this form of medicine tends to be more associated with the present day inheritors of public health. In Great Britain and Ireland the specialty is known as Community Medicine and the practitioners as Community Physicians. It may help to clarify discussion, if an attempt is made to distinguish some of the more common terms used to describe the sciences of disease control and health promotion.

Public Health

As the term is now used the emphasis is on the protection and promotion of the health of the total population through legislation and by social action at local and central government levels. Control of health hazards in the physical environment is emphasized.

Community Medicine

This is a branch of medicine concerned with the health care of groups and communities, through the application of epidemiology and medical care organization.

Preventive Medicine

This logically is a branch of medicine but is sometimes used more broadly. It tends to be administered more personally than in Public Health. Physicians and health services aim at a more clinical level to carry out health education, vaccination and screening for disease.

Social Medicine

While sharing the broad aims of the other disciplines, social medicine tends also to be concerned with the social aspects of the clinical case (occupation, behaviour) and with group living as a factor in health and disease.

JUSTIFICATION FOR PREVENTION

Survival of the herd is perhaps the most fundamental objective of society. As life and wellbeing are attributes closely associated with survival, it might be concluded that their value was a 'self-evident truth'. It might be further argued that preventing pain, disability and premature death require no justification. This perspective sees life and health as either good in themselves or as desirable second level objectives.

The reality, however, is that individuals are unimportant to herd survival, and in practice the promotion of health cannot be achieved without cost, effort or resources, bringing it into conflict with competing demands, and compelling the 'value of life' to take its turn in the list of social priorities.

The superiority of prevention as an alternative strategy in maintaining life and health is a widely held belief—an ounce of prevention is worth a pound of cure. As implied by the proverb, measures taken to avert disease tend to be relatively simple and inexpensive. Preventive measures, if effective, would also be humane, because the pain, suffering and disability which would have occurred have been averted. A third element in the belief is that much illness is not effectively curable. These generalizations are probably reasonably valid. Much evaluation of this nature has been carried out and still continues. Epidemiological studies give, for example, the cost of a positive case detected in screening surveys. If, for example, such a figure should be £10 000 who is to decide if this is too much?

There is a view that, irrespective of cost, prevention is intrinsically superior in itself. This was expressed by Lord Milner in his frequently quoted assertion (26 November 1909): 'If we believe a thing to be bad, and if we have a right to prevent it, it is our duty to try to prevent it and to damn the consequences'.

OBSTACLES TO PREVENTION

Prevention tends to be highly regarded in theory but neglected in practice. Only a small percentage of total expenditure on medical care goes to further health promotion or disease prevention. The reasons for this are complex and include social and cultural attitudes, as well as economic and ethical factors. In addition the issues and concepts will be seen differently as between the general public, the preventive care providers and the government.

There is a common tendency for people to be more concerned with the concrete immediacy of the present than with the possibilities of the future. Maturation of the human personality expands time-consciousness from the tendency to live in the extended present towards a greater awareness of the past and at the same time an ability to take account of the future. In so far as prevention emphasizes what will not happen in the future it is a negative concept which will inevitably increase difficulties in persuasion. While thinkers in the field of health promotion are well aware of these and other obstacles in influencing community health, it is still true that many campaigns could be rendered ineffective because of lack of awareness among interventionists of the factors governing health behaviours. One factor described is the 'fallacy of the empty vessel'[11]—that is, the assumption that the general public is empty of health knowledge and that it is a matter of filling the vessel with information. The fallacy is that people already have their own established health customs and beliefs. It is suggested that professional workers, to be effective, must know and respect the culture of their population. Further attempts to understand why there may be resistance to preventive health advice have led to the construction of what is described as the health belief model (HBM).[12] The theory outlines the following factors as influencing a person's preventive behaviour: (1) general concern about health matters; (2) perceived susceptibility of acquiring a particular disease or disorder; (3) perceived seriousness of a risked disease or disorder; (4) perceived benefits to be realized by engaging in particular preventive behaviour, as opposed to the costs of such behaviour or actions; and (5) cues to action—that is, information or advice that focusses the attention of the individual on specific preventive behaviour.

While the model has provided an understanding of the use of certain preventive medical services such as immunization and screening programmes,[11] it is essentially confined to factors within the individual, and appears to assume that each individual is a free agent with a large range of behavioural options at his disposal. From the point of view of public health, however, many behaviour patterns are socially, culturally and economically determined, and are not simply the result of individual free choice. For many, a healthy diet may be achieved only at great cost or inconvenience and for others smoking and drinking to excess may be closely related to social pressures. Furthermore, the individual is powerless to change factors in the physical environment.

Nevertheless creating an atmosphere which would enhance the social value of prevention requires cooperative effort between the citizens and government. The state will only act to pass public health legislation if such measures are acceptable to the population, because each measure is a further restriction of liberty. In the light of the great amount of road safety legislation that has been passed without objection in most countries it seems clear that the public is more likely to accept these types of restrictions on individual autonomy than other types of preventive measures such as fluoridation of drinking water. At the same time it appears that legislative authority, once exerted, can in itself produce population acquiescence virtually overnight, one of the best examples being the chlorination of water.

The view is sometimes expressed that prevention is good in theory but when you get down to it, it is often very impractical or politically impossible. This is a way of saying that the economic, political or social costs of prevention are too great. This view may be contrasted with the huge sums of money often spent on a single case under treatment. The human drama of the individual case can move total populations to exceptional limits of generosity. A radio appeal in Ireland raised £1 million to send a boy to the United States for a liver transplant. In contrast, thousand of deaths tend to be regarded as just statistics. This human perspective of the disease problem provides a challenge to the promoters of public health.

The successful objectives of prevention have no drama, because saved lives are non-events. The persons whose lives have been saved have no identity. It is rare even for preventive services to publish regular statistics of the number of cases averted or of lives saved. As a corollary, it is very difficult to single out those who have been responsible for saving lives. Equally difficult is the identification of those who may have been negligent in prevention. Part of the explanation is that fatalism about disease is common even among health care professionals. The spirit of fatalism is contrary to preventive efforts because it is based either on a theory of the intrinsic randomness of disease or on the influence of forces beyond human control.

Reference has been made to popular attitudes as an important factor in the promotion of preventive measures. It is frequently made difficult for the population to understand the purpose of prevention. Some are of the view that they are being encouraged to extend the normal life-span; others think that the educators are interested only in some diseases and not others. Therefore it is common to hear 'one has to die of something'. Prevention can sometimes be seen as threatening and the perceived or actual adverse effects of intervention, as in the case of whooping cough, awaken much greater concern than the side-effects of drugs given for treatment.

Some of these obstacles arise out of the essential nature of prevention, and others relate to aspects of current practice. In an ideal society which was much more committed to preventive measures than we are at present very few of the obstacles would prove insuperable.

REFERENCES

1. Wain, H. *A History of Preventive Medicine*. Springfield, Illinois: Charles C. Thomas, 1970: 7–11.
2. Castliglioni, A. *A History of Medicine*. Second edition. New York: Alfred A. Knopf, 1958: 901.
3. Frank, J. P. *System einer vollständigen medicinischen Polizei*. Nine volumes. Mannheim Tübingen, Wien; 1779–1827.
4. Duncan, A. *A Short View of the Extent and Importance of Medical Jurisprudence as a Branch of Education*. Edinburgh: Edinburgh University, 1806.
5. Blaney, R. Henry Maunsell (1807–1879): an early community physician. *Ir J Med Sci* 1984; **153**: 42–43.
6. Haddon, W. Advances in the epidemiology of injuries as a basis for public policy. *Public Health Rep* 1980; **95**: 411–421.
7. Susser, M. *Causal Thinking in the Health Sciences*. New York: Oxford University Press, 1973.
8. Hospers, J. *An Introduction to Philosophical Analysis*. London: Routledge and Kegan Paul, 1978.
9. Clark, D. W. and MacMahon, B. *Preventive and Community Medicine*. Second edition. Boston: Little, Brown and Company, 1981: 7.

10. Last, J. M. (ed). *A Dictionary of Epidemiology*. Handbook sponsored by the International Epidemiological Association. New York: Oxford University Press, 1983.
11. Levine, S. and Sorenson, J. R. Social and cultural factors in health promotion. Chapter 14. **In**: Matarazzo *et al.* (eds). *Behavioural Health: a Handbook of Health Enhancement and Disease Prevention*. New York: John Wiley & Sons, 1984.
12. Becker, M. Psychosocial aspects of health related behaviour. **In**: Freeman, H., Levine, S. and Reeder, L. (eds). *Handbook of Medical Sociology*. Third edition. Englewood Cliffs, NJ: Prentice-Hall, 1979.

PART B

POLICIES AND GENERAL PROBLEMS

Ethical Dilemmas in Health Promotion
Edited by S. Doxiadis

CHAPTER 6

Personal and Public Health Care: Conflict, Congruence or Accommodation?

E. G. KNOX

SUMMARY

Contrasts are drawn between the work of doctors engaged in personal practice, and those providing a service to the population. Differences in style and in objectives lead occasionally to conflict. We then distinguish between false and true conflicts. False conflicts arise from muddled thinking, or sometimes by intention. They can be resolved through analysis and argument. The question arises whether the conflict between personal and population practice is false in this sense, or whether it has deeper origins. Four separate illustrations—rationing, fluoridation, vaccination and the confidentiality of medical records—suggest a genuine and indelible conflict, not capable of resolution through formal argument. Possible solutions based upon appeal to higher principles such as 'justice', the 'right to privacy', or the 'right to self-determination', are examined. They fail to resolve the conflict. Our actions must be guided by the principle of *minimizing* moral damage, rather than *eliminating* it altogether.

CONTRASTS OF STYLE

Doctors engaged in personal consulting practice—both general and specialist—and those responsible for developing preventive and therapeutic services at the population level, share broad objectives and common ethics. Modern reformulations of the Hippocratic oath emphasize their joint concern both for individuals and for mankind. Despite the modern epidemic of restrictive job-descriptions, many practitioners in each of these fields contribute substantially to the other.

There is however a contrast of style and of priorities. The *first* concern of the clinical doctor is the patient before him; whereas the *first* concern of the community physician is the good of the population as a whole. The object of the clinical doctor's concern is an *identified* person; while the 'patients' of the community physician are not necessarily identifiable. Where preventive services are concerned, he hopes they never will be.

These contrasts lead occasionally to difficulties and even to conflict. The purpose of this chapter is to examine the nature of these collisions. Are they real conflicts? Do they arise inevitably from the pursuit of different objectives? Are they rather the product of human fallibility? Can they be avoided? How can they be accommodated when they occur?

CONFLICTS OF INTEREST

False Antitheses and False Conflicts

Sir Douglas Black pursued the theme of false conflict in his recent Rock Carling monograph *An Anthology of False Antitheses*.[1] He used the term 'false' in two separate senses—some antitheses are false in not being antitheses at all; and some are also false in intention, having been engineered to create conflict where none truly exists.

For example, the opposition of the 'medical model' and the 'social model' of illness serves the useful function of characterizing different perceptions of sickness; but many doctors will have been surprised to learn that their own perceptions are as strictly limited as some have suggested. The contrast between 'holistic' and 'allopathic' medicine is still a mystery to them. When they read to their surprise that they practise only the latter, that they are taught to treat diseases rather than patients, and that they are incapable of dealing with patients 'as a whole', they begin to suspect that someone is grinding axes. And so they are. The purpose of such denigration is to alter the general balance of professional esteem.

[It is standard practice in such Pecking Order Games, first to pronounce a false premise, then attach it to the victim, and finally knock it down. If all goes well, the victim comes down heavily with the false premise. There is no good pithy English word for this process. 'Aunt Sally-ism' is clumsy. 'Petitio Principii'—from the dictionaries—is opaque. If we had a good technical term analogous with the 'Double Question' (When did you stop beating your wife?), we might be able to deal with it more effectively.]

As part of his analysis, Sir Douglas goes on to say that he believes the contrast between population and personal medicine is a false antithesis in this mould. The conflicts are between the professionals, and not between their 'customers'. Populations are simply the sums of the individuals within them, so why *should* there be a problem? What is good for populations is good for individuals; what is good for individuals is good for populations.

But is this really true? Let us look at four concrete problems.

Rationing

The medical world is characterized—perhaps for ever—by over-demand and limited resource. The original objective of the National Health Service in Britain was to make all necessary medical care available without charge at the point of demand. Rudolf Klein has argued persuasively that the process has gone into reverse.[2] According to his analysis, a main attraction of a centrally financed service, such as the National Health Service, seen through political eyes, is that through ensuring a reasonable degree of equity, it makes scarcity acceptable. The maintenance of scarcity, permitting limitation of expenditure, has thus become one of its *de facto* objectives. It has become a rationing system and, like it or not, doctors working in the field of public health are involved in the operation of a restrictive process. This brings them into conflict with clinical doctors, whose duty on behalf of their patients, is to demand *more*.

On more detailed examination, however, it appears that the clinicians are also involved in this rationing process. The conflict is 'tactical' rather than fundamental. Both groups are involved in distributing resources to those who depend upon them, while at the same time trying to extract resources from those on whom they depend. The clinical doctor rations his time between his patients while trying to attract resources from the Health Authority, while the Community Physicians and the Management Teams distribute available resources between different specialties and different institutions and different client groups, while trying to obtain more from Senior Authorities, or from the government. The positions of the two specialty groups within this chain differ, but both are engaged in the common process of transmitting pressures from patients to politicians, and vice versa. They work, still, within a common ethical system, and their different locations within the chain of pressure provide no grounds for tearing our profession apart.

However, if doctors are not in fundamental conflict with each other, then it is equally clear that within a non-explicit rationing system, each individual competes with the rest of the community. Indeed, if we resolve this to its particular elements, each individual competes with every other.

Fluoridation

A relationship between mottled teeth and local water supplies was known in the last century. The connection with fluoride was discovered later and, in the 1930s, an association was noted between dental mottling and low levels of dental caries. The connection between fluoride and caries prevention was subsequently inferred both in the United States and in England (at Malden in Essex). During the 1940s in the United States, and during the 1950s in the United Kingdom, planned intervention experiments of drinking water fluoridation were carried out, treated areas being matched with control areas, and the protective effect was confirmed. The experimental populations were monitored for ill-effects and, as in the natural high fluoride areas, no evidence of harm was found. The true nature of a number of hypochondriacal reactions to fluoridation was readily demonstrated through the doubtfully ethical trick of postponing fluoridation until after the predeclared date. Reports from Canada,[3–5] which suggested an association with Down's Syndrome, caused some alarm but were shown to be based upon faulty data and incompetent analysis. Firm positive reassurance on this particular point, and in relation to other congenital malformations has since been obtained in Birmingham which was fluoridated in 1964.[6]

More recently, there have been repeated allegations of a cancer hazard both in the United States and in the United Kingdom. These allegations came essentially from two workers who stand almost alone against all other scientific opinion. A Working Party of the Royal College of Physicians in 1976,[7] and a more recent one set up by the Secretary of State for Health, and reporting in 1985[8] concluded that all the associations alleged by these workers could be traced to faulty data or faulty analysis or faulty reasoning, or a combination of all three. Other Commissions in other places have come to the same conclusion. Competent analyses of natural variation of fluoride and of artificial fluoridation in a wide range of circumstances in many different countries have provided very substantial positive reassurance that this measure is safe.

Nevertheless, a legitimate issue remains. A small group of people continue to object to supplementation of the fluoride levels of their drinking water in the manner recommended. The demonstratable scientific falsity of the allegations of harm which have often accompanied their objections, the mischievous ways in which the claims were pressed, and the fact that similar objections have been deployed in the past in relation to other life-saving proposals, such as smallpox vaccination, seat-belts, crash helmets, make no difference. The unavoidable fact is that if we are to implement this public health measure then it is necessary that the majority overrides the wishes of the minority. The alternative is that the minority overrides the wishes of the majority. There is nothing which will make this confrontation go away, or which will allow us to evade the necessity of making the decision. Individual objectors are in conflict with a society which fluoridates. Individual sufferers are in conflict with one which does not.

Vaccination

If a doctor is asked his opinion about whooping-cough vaccination in a particular child, with a specific question about the risk, his best advice might be that the parents should try to arrange that their child is the only unvaccinated one in the community. He gets protection without risk. However, this is not advice which can be given to everyone.

The principle embedded in this ridiculous example finds a serious though inverted application in the design of policies to eradicate Congenital Rubella Syndrome

(CRS). Rubella vaccine benefits those to whom it is given—or rather their children. In contrast to the whooping-cough example, however, it actually harms those to whom it is not given. It does this by interfering with the normal transmission of the disease, and postponing the age at natural infection among the unvaccinated part of the population. This increases the proportion of unvaccinated girls reaching child-bearing age without the natural immunity which they might otherwise have received. One group loses while the other group gains. The net effect in the population as a whole is the balance of the beneficial and harmful effects.

In countries such as the United Kingdom, where vaccination is offered in adolescence only to girls, so that there is little effect upon the transmission of Rubella, the harmful effects are limited. In programmes such as that adopted in the United States, where the vaccine is given to young children of both sexes, high levels of uptake will eliminate the virus and, with it, the Congenital Rubella Syndrome. The benefits are high, but so are the risks. If eradication is *not* achieved, the risk to the unvaccinated fraction is substantial. In some circumstances, a failed eradication programme will cause more cases of CRS than it prevents.[9,10]

The theory of predicting the effects of alternative policies is well worked out. The American method would be superior in the United Kingdom if over 90 per cent of the population were immunized and if this proportion could be maintained, while the current British method is superior (in the long term) if the best that can be achieved is about a 75 per cent uptake. Either policy is better than no policy—like driving on the left or driving on the right. The worst possible situation is to have no policy at all. For example, I heard the policy of one South American country defined as—'our policy is that you buy the vaccine from the chemist and ask your doctor to give it'.

The ethical problem is that the most effective and most rapidly acting policy, aimed at eradication, requires either compulsion or else a remarkable degree of persuasion, to attain and maintain the necessary level of uptake. If such compulsion is not accepted, then it is the wrong policy. The risks are just too great. We would then do better to accept this and to choose the less efficient system—as we have in fact done in the United Kingdom—accepting *some* loss of life deliberately rather than pressing on in ill-judged hope, and incurring a subsequent *large* loss of life. Either way, we must choose a policy and then impose it—that is, the wishes of some individuals must be overridden. Eradication requires compulsion. Compulsion is a manifestation of conflict between the society and the individual.

In countries where there is no firm policy of any kind, or no means of implementing it, or where there is a regionally divided policy, the clinical doctor is in a difficult position. His advice must be to vaccinate in order to protect his patients from the consequences of the administrative chaos. It will worry him to know that for every case of CRS he saves, he might be causing two;

but he has no real choice. The casualties will probably be someone else's patients, and he will never know their names.

Confidentiality of Medical Records and Their Use in Research

The Hippocratic Oath is no longer formally taken, and its strictures on abortion have been cast rather lightly aside, but its declared principle of secrecy is still followed; apart, that is, from a few exceptions. Regular or occasional access to medical information is now acceded to other doctors, secretaries, records officers, computer staff, administrators, statisticians, research workers, armed forces authorities, the Registrar of Births, Deaths and Marriages, and courts of law. The permissible uses of medical records are also very closely defined by professional organizations. They are said to be purely for the benefit of the patient in the course of his or her medical care. Once more, however, there is a list of exceptions. They are used for costing, managing the institutions in which care is given, compiling service activity statistics, pursuing research and protecting doctors and institutions against litigation.

This pattern of a strictly stated containment, both in terms of purpose and of person, but with an extended set of exceptions, has been adopted almost everywhere. Plainly, it is double-think. The list of exceptions is now so extensive as to be almost open-ended, and it is impossible to control the release of information beyond the first stage. As a matter of operational fact, the regulatory defences of secrecy are ineffective, and we rely entirely upon the good sense of individual doctors and of other health workers.

Attempts to control these problems through regulatory means have followed different pathways in different countries. In Britain, the medium on which the record is written belongs to the Secretary of State for Health, and the doctor is regarded as the guardian or custodian of the content. In Gallic countries, where the genitive case is interpreted differently, the 'patients' record is treated as if it belonged, literally, to the patient. In Scandinavian countries, state finance of the health system renders a medical record a sub-class of 'public' record. With their tradition of openness, public records are generally accessible to anyone! Needless to say a patchwork of *ad hoc* regulation has been developed in each location to prevent the worst abuses of literal interpretation. The Scandinavians have so managed their affairs that people are *not* allowed to look at other peoples' records. The French have managed theirs so that doctors are allowed to keep them on their files. In practice, and no matter from which original standpoint the legislation *began*, we have all ended up with much the same working system.

The only real casualty so far has been research, or rather the future patients whose welfare depends upon this research. Those without scientific or medical training often fail to recognize that *everything* which we know has been learned through research, that we are totally dependent upon it for the development of health care, and that without it we will learn nothing more. Much of it is dependent upon the release and use of medical records. Unfortunately, the non-comprehending non-scientists include some legislators, and where their brief covers social legislation relating to all kinds of records, and not just medical records, there is more than a possibility that the proper consideration of research requirements is simply mislaid.

I was Chairman of a Working Group of the Commission of the European Communities examining these problems, and attempting to define rules of usage and access in a positive manner, encompassed within a code of practice.[11] We tried to be realistic, declaring the boundaries of usage and access in a manner which might then be truly enforced, in contrast with the customary practice of declaring limits in an unrealistic style, necessitating a consequent growth of unadmitted open-ended leaks. For this it is necessary not only to consider the interests of the individual about whom the record is written, but the interests of *all* patients and potential patients, present and future.

The problem is that the good of the community depends upon each person individually relinquishing something which in the past has sometimes been stated as an absolute right. Once more, therefore, we identify conflict between person and people, and between this person and that person, for which there can be no formal solution. Strict reliance upon the principle of the public good, and strict reliance upon the principle of personal rights, are each equally untenable. In this example, as in the earlier ones, the problem of conflict between individual and society simply will not go away.

GUIDING PRINCIPLES

Ubiquity of Ethical Conflict

Most of us are by now used to the idea of rationing scarce resources, and recognize that doctors are involved in this process. If it is recommended that this woman should have a cervical smear *every* year, then another will get less than she needs, or else the time spent by the microscopist upon each smear will be reduced, and the sensitivity of the test will fall. If one patient gets 10 minutes in the surgery, then another will get only two. Demand, supply and standards of care, must be traded off against each other. If the supply is for the time being fixed, then one of the other two must give. Rationing by price, or rationing by waiting list, or rationing by standard: different methods—but rationing all the same.

We are also well used to the idea, formulated if not discovered by the sociologists, that the outcomes expected from a medical consultation differ as between doctor and patient; there is sometimes a conflict of purpose, perhaps exacerbated by poor communication, even in this central relationship.

However, we see both of these problems imposed by special circumstances (for example, shortages) or by human frailty (for example, stupidity, inadequate understanding, and so on). The idea that some conflicts might arise from *neither* of these sources, and that they might be inevitable, inescapable and unresolvable, is at first more difficult to stomach. Yet, as the examples show, the joint concern of medicine for the good of the individual and for the good of mankind—as stated clearly in the Geneva Convention—does in a number of concrete situations bring patient into conflict with population; or, to resolve it into its elements, one person into conflict with another.

The idea of an unresolvable conflict and of inherent inconsistency is a difficult one for scientists, and perhaps also for legislators. Legislators and lawyers are of course familiar with conflict, but they work on the general premiss that it can be resolved through the application of a set of rules and principles, at least to the reasonable satisfaction of society, if not necessarily of the parties. Scientists do not normally permit themselves the softening effects of this last clause; with respect to conflict, they work in absolutes. That is, they work from the premiss that the material world is consistent, and that any demonstrated lack of consistency is a reflection upon the evidence or the argument that went into the demonstration. Consistency is the primary axiom of their world. The scientific and logical elements of the professional training of doctors and lawyers provide little guidance for handling so formally intractable a problem as balancing the good of the individual against the good of his fellows. It is perhaps for these reasons that we find our public health services in such disarray at the present time, and so lacking in resources, professional esteem, or even a proper allocation of professional responsibilities. Even the *ethics* of public health programmes and research are regularly set in a very firm second place to the ethics of the medical consultation; if such ethics are fortunate enough to be recognized at all!

Solutions Based on Higher Principles

Rawls, in his *Theory of Justice*,[12] tried to tackle some of these problems. His general proposal (slightly parodied) is that social policies involving redistributions of benefit, can be considered 'just' only when no harm befalls the least-advantaged member of the society. However, it is difficult to see how this principle could be applied successfully to some of the examples quoted. Harm befalls the least advantaged for any decision whatever, including no decision. Rawls' dictum seems to be designed for situations where the benefits, the disbenefits and the people, and the connections between specific benefits and particular individuals, can each be identified in advance. It is less clearly appropriate for a redistribution of *risk*, with nothing quite so specific as an identified beneficiary.

Within its proper field of application, Rawls' proposition appeals to a higher principle, namely 'justice'. There are other 'higher principles' from which to choose, and they include the so-called 'fundamental human rights'. In relation to confidentiality, the 'right' in question is 'privacy'. The right to privacy has been defined as follows: 'Every one has the right to respect for his privacy and family life, his home and his correspondence. There shall be no interference by a public Authority with the exercise of this right except such as is in accordance with the law and is necessary in a democratic society in the interests of national security, public safety or the economic wellbeing of the country, for the prevention of disorder or crime, for the protection of health or morals, or for the protection of the rights and freedom of others'.

It starts well enough, but soon begins to read like Orwell. The problem with this approach is that the 'right' is conferred by society, and when we encounter a circumstance in which the maintenance of the right threatens the existence of the society, the declaration becomes inconsistent and non-self-sustaining. There appears to be no escape, at least along these lines, from the conflict between population and person.

Similar problems arise in relation to compulsory health measures such as vaccination and fluoridation. The 'right' in question here, and the one in danger of being infringed, is the 'right to self-determination'. Any definition encounters the same kind of problem. The society which confers the rights must be protected in order to have an opportunity of conferring them! The exceptions necessary for this protection themselves infringe the 'right'. The notion of a 'right' begins to lose the commonly attached attributes of being 'fundamental', or 'inviolable', or 'absolute'. It becomes simply a desirable state of affairs.

No Way Out?

At least in the field of public and personal health, we must probably accept that if the rights of the individual are supported to the exclusion of all else, then the society which provides the protection is at hazard. And this means its individual members. However, if the rights of the society are enforced to the exclusion of all else, then the willingness of individuals to be part of that society is diminished. Absolute sovereignty of the one over the other, in either direction, has to be rejected. We must probably work towards a pragmatic solution, rather than one which can be justified in formally argued terms. Practical solutions will probably take the form of a 'code of practice', which seeks to minimize moral damage, rather than to eliminate it altogether.

The development and formulation of *detailed* practical 'solutions' is a task for another occasion—although the path is perhaps exemplified in the EEC Report on Confidentiality. This is not the objective of the present chapter. Its objective is rather to *identify* the indelible nature of the problem. If we are to learn how to deal with it effectively then we must not pretend that it does not exist, or suppose that a little legislation is all that is needed to tidy it up.

REFERENCES

1. Black, D. *An Anthology of False Antitheses*. The Rock Carling Fellowship. London: Nuffield Provincial Hospitals Trust, 1984.
2. Klein, R. *The Politics of the National Health Service*. Harlow: Longman, 1984.
3. Rapaport, I. Contributions to the study of Mongolism. The pathogenic role of fluorine. *Bull Acad Nat Med (Paris)* 1956; **140**: 528–531.
4. Rapaport, I. New Research on Mongolism. The Pathogenic role of fluorine. *Bull Acad Nat Med (Paris)* 1959; **143**: 367–370.
5. Rapaport, I. Mongol Oligophrenia and Dental Caries. *Rev Stomatol (Paris)* 1963; **46**: 207–218.
6. Knox, E. G., Armstrong, E. and Lancashire R. Fluoridation and the prevalence of congenital malformations. *Community Medicine* 1980; **2**: 190–194.
7. Royal College of Physicians. *Fluoride, Teeth and Health*. London: Pitmans, 1976.
8. *Report of the Working Party on Fluoridation of Water and Cancer: A review of the Epidemiological Evidence*. London: Her Majesty's Stationery Office, 1985.
9. Knox, E. G. Strategy for Rubella Vaccination. *Int J Epidemiol* 1980; **9**: 13–23.
10. Knox, E. G. Theoretical aspects of rubella vaccination strategies. *Int J Infect Dis* 1984; **7**: 194–197.
11. *The Confidentiality of Medical Records. The Principles and Practice of Protection in a Research-Dependent Environment*. Report EUR 9471 EN. Brussels and Luxembourg: Commission of the European Communities, 1984.
12. Rawls, J. *A Theory of Justice*. Oxford: Clarendon Press 1973.

Ethical Dilemmas in Health Promotion
Edited by S. Doxiadis

CHAPTER 7

Life-Style, Public Health and Paternalism

DAN BEAUCHAMP

SUMMARY

The number of health problems associated with voluntary risks is very large. The question of whether government should resort to paternalistic legislation such as limits to drinking, smoking, or using the motor car is central. Many commentators are strict antipaternalists, or accept paternalism only very grudgingly. I would argue that paternalism to protect the public health is not only compatible with democratic values, but that types of paternalism, like public health restrictions, are essential to defend the common life and to promote a sense of community. Moreover, a strict antipaternalism is hard to maintain, and the clamour for action often results in measures to promote health and safety focused unfairly and ineffectually on certain groups in society, such as the young or those believed to be mostly responsible for health problems. Another reason why public health paternalism is justified is that it is minimally intrusive to individuals, since it consists mainly of controls placed on the market place or the use of market goods in the public realm. Finally, while public health paternalism does involve restrictions on private liberty, the ends of such paternalistic restrictions are shared and collective in nature, not private ones, and promote group virtues like beneficence and concern for the common good.

INTRODUCTION

In recent decades it has become a truism that a significant portion (perhaps as much as half) of the disease and early death in industrialized societies stems from personal risk-taking. Dealing with these risks—commonly called life-style risks—creates substantial political difficulties in democratic societies.

Questions of what to do about cigarette smoking, alcohol use, or driving without seat-belts arouse great political debate. Policy restrictions for life-style choices have in Western democracies been influenced by a strong antipaternalism.

Antipaternalism flourishes in many conditions, but its native soil is political individualism. Political individualism assumes that the political community is an association of self-determining individuals who view the 'purpose of government as confined to enabling individuals' wants to be satisfied, individuals' interests to be pursued and individuals' rights to be protected, with a clear bias toward *laissez-faire* and against the idea that [the government] might legitimately influence or alter their wants, interpret their interests for them or invade or abrogate their rights'.[1]

Many would protest that most Western democracies are today far removed from political individualism. This is clearly true—the exception remains the United States. Nevertheless, a strong antipaternalism characterizes the European welfare states with the notable exception of many of the Nordic countries. This antipaternalism flourishes because the growth of the welfare state has been justified in terms of a vision of equality that is ambiguous on the idea of whether society should only enable individuals to pursue their own ends or should pursue common ends. The ideas of justice and equality found in the post-World War 2 Welfare State were often based on loosening government restrictions on personal life outside the economic sphere, partly as a concession to the new found power of the working class, who had been the most common target of restrictive policies, such as prohibition.[2]

PATERNALISM VERSUS ANTIPATERNALISM

Moving away from antipaternalism to a democracy that includes some forms of paternalism, especially for public health, does not imply political collectivism or the view that government seeks only to improve the welfare of the community and that the citizenry have only loyalties to the larger interests of society. Democracy that includes some legitimate forms of paternalism is based on the view that government must reconcile two main ends: the rights and interests of the individual taken separately and the good of individuals together—the community—even for life-style risks.

In a democracy which seeks to reconcile and balance the good of the individual with the good of the whole, a chief purpose of public policy is to cope with what Brian Barry calls the standard liberal fallacy: the fallacy that what is in the interest of the individual is also in the interest of the community.[3] This conflict is felt most acutely in the private market-place where health and safety concerns are not sufficiently protected, but the gap is also present in the public economy, such as in the provision of medical care under national insurance schemes. While this view of democracy does not challenge the idea that the purpose of government is to promote the welfare of individuals, democracy as dialectic assumes that we as a society are *both* a collection of private individuals and groups and also a political community pursuing common ends and a common life.

In a democracy based on both community and paternalism to protect the public health, as well as individual autonomy, government seeks to reconcile individual virtues like self-reliance and individual responsibility with community virtues like beneficence, cooperation, and justice.[4] Beneficence means that we wish the good and welfare of others as well as ourselves, while cooperation and justice mean that we as citizens are disposed to see that the common welfare is extended to all alike and do not allow our private interests to frustrate achievement of the common good. While the principles of individuality and community can often pull in opposite directions, both principles are needed to assure the fullest development of the individual and his dignity both as an autonomous person and as a member of the political fellowship.

The backbone of antipaternalism is the harm principle as captured in John Stuart Mill's famous essay *On Liberty*.[5] '[T]he only purpose for which power can be rightfully exercised over any member of a civilised community, against his will, is to prevent harm to others'. According to Mill, the state cannot legitimately require the individual to take care for his own safety, and self-regarding faults are not properly immoralities. They may be proofs of any amount of folly, or want of personal dignity and self-respect; but they are only a subject of moral reprobation when they involve a breach of duty to others, for whose sake the individual is bound to have care for himself. What are called duties to ourselves are not socially obligatory unless circumstances render them at the same time duties to others.

In Mill's scheme, regulating unhealthy or risky behaviour among autonomous adults can only be to prevent specific wrongs that one group visits on another, or because judgment or action is seriously impaired. In this view, drunk driving would be a public problem; alcoholism pure and simple would not—'Drunkenness . . . in ordinary cases is not a fit subject for legislative interference . . . '.[5] Others would expand Mill's individualism by extending the range of effects which individual acts are said to cause, and by enlarging the duties of individuals to others. Thus, smokers and drinkers would be made directly liable for the increased costs they might place on the medical care system, under the theory that their voluntary acts do cause injury to others. Similarly those who drive without seat-belts may be said to increase the costs of medical care, and can be charged higher premiums, or even denied all or part of their insurance claims.

Antipaternalists recognize the need for collective goods and that this requires often serious restrictions on liberty. Collective goods are goods which because of features of 'jointness' or 'non-excludability' are undersupplied in market economies and must be provided under government intervention. Most antipaternalists allow a broader range of restrictions on private liberty to provide for collective protections like defence, fire and police protection, and a common legal system. Preventive measures to improve health, such as air and water pollution control, are often justified as nonpaternalistic because private actions alone cannot bring them into being. For example, it is impossible to fluoridate and chlorinate the water supply for only those individuals who desire treated water; hence, the need for universal protection. Likewise, if a majority wants protection against industrial pollution or smog from car exhausts, the entire society must be protected because of the joint nature of the preventive measure itself.

In the view of democracy as permitting more paternalistic interventions to strike a better balance between community and the freedom of the individual, the collective goods argument is crucial. Indeed, the failure of markets and private arrangements to provide collective goods is the principal reason and justification for community organization. Schelling calls this conflict between the individual and the common good the 'summing-up problem',[6] and Hirsch describes it as 'choice in the small' versus 'choice in the large';[7] both express the view that the good of each of us is not the same thing as the good of all of us together. Collective goods are not simply commodities which the market cannot provide in the community; they are not commodities at all. Collective goods are ultimately a set of relationships among the citizens of a community, relationships in which the community as a whole participates to obtain desired benefits. These collective goods include aggregate states of welfare or wellbeing, including declining rates of disease and premature deaths; efforts to limit the resources society devotes to providing personal health services; shared and common access to a good like medical care to foster the sense of community and membership in the group itself. And finally, there are those highly important collective goods, shared or common beliefs and values.

Among the Western democracies, the United States has more than any other embraced a philosophy of political individualism. Yet even in the United States there has always been a distinct tradition of balancing individualism with community interests, both in theory and in practice. The Puritans were not rugged individualists; their communitarian principles are found in the early New England constitutions.[8] The development of the state powers to regulate private property for the common good—what are usually called the regulatory or police powers—are not limited to 'Sic utere tuo ut alienum non laedas' ('So use your property as not to injure the property of others'), the common law and Roman antecedents of the harm principle.[9] The Courts have consistently given legislatures the power to fluoridate and chlorinate the common water system, to require cyclists to wear helmets, to make vaccination compulsory, and even to permit complete state prohibition of alcohol.[10]

THE CASE OF ALCOHOL PROBLEMS

In the remainder of this chapter I wish to examine the consequences of antipaternalism and the balancing approach for limiting life-style risks, focussing mainly on alcohol problems and policy. Alcohol problems, given the long history of alcohol regulation in political communities, offer a vehicle for examining the issues in complex life-style questions. My thesis is that balancing group and private interests offer a more adequate framework for life-style risks and avoid some of the pitfalls of antipaternalism. I argue that public health paternalism has three advantages over antipaternalism.

Firstly, public health paternalism encourages us to confront how the organization of the market place and the world of trade and commerce affects the level of life-style risks in the community. The changing structure of the market has baleful influences on hazards like smoking or drinking just as this structure also influences the level of more involuntary risks like unemployment, pollution, or consumer fraud.

Secondly, public health paternalism provides many benefits beyond improving individual welfare—benefits like the community virtues of cooperation and mutual dependence. Up to a point, there is even reason to believe that paternalism may also strengthen individual independence and autonomy.

Thirdly, public health paternalism may protect individual and private interests better than antipaternalism. Antipaternalism often results in policies that put too much emphasis on fixing blame, or on restrictions for youth, or on even more extreme measures like prohibition.

The Structural Side of Alcohol Problems

What has been the experience of the Western democracies with alcohol problems in the post-war period? With the exception of France, the general experience has been that alcohol consumption in the aggregate has increased greatly, reflecting the fundamental increase in economic productivity and personal consumption that occurred in the decades from 1950s to the 1970s.[11] Alcohol became, during this period, a commodity much like others. Community sanctions over alcohol commerce were gradually but dramatically weakened in many places. Alcohol products like beer became available in general retail outlet chains, which themselves greatly expanded. Regional and local restrictions were relaxed or totally eliminated. The hours of sale expanded. Age limits were often reduced. Drinking patterns became increasingly homogeneous across national and regional boundaries. Advertising and other forms of promotion dramatically increased.

Given these developments, it should come as no surprise that drinking increased—as did alcohol problems. What is surprising is that while alcohol consumption and consequent problems increased, until very recently governments did not strengthen their alcohol control efforts. This lack of action was the result of many factors, as Christie[2] and others[11] have noted. The post-World War 2 period was one of sharply increasing economic productivity, urban growth, and a shift from traditional values of hard work, thrift, and abstemiousness to modernist values like consumerism, liberation from communal restraints, and leisure. Also, the egalitarian ethos of the welfare state was a mixture of growing supervision of economic life and of spreading welfare systems, with a loosening of restrictions on personal life.[11] Political individualism was on the wane in the economic sphere but it was on the rise in the personal sphere.

The post-war growth of the welfare state and the treatment professions brought with it a commitment to expanded treatment resources for the sick alcoholic; alcohol control policies were often associated with punishment and maltreatment of the alcoholic. Temperance forces declined in political influence in many countries. Also, as I have already mentioned, alcohol control policies were often perceived as controls on the working class, and post-war welfare policies were enacted in part because of the increased political power of the working class.[11] Finally, the economic interests of the producer groups solidified and were strengthened during this period.

Thus a paradox arose: just as alcohol problems and drinking were on the rise in Western societies, many governments were abandoning their commitments to alcohol control. The major exception to this pattern has been drunk driving.[11]

One of forces countering this trend has been the growing influence of public health agencies and public health interests in society. The new public health, and the 'second epidemiological revolution'[12] that undergirds it, call attention not only to the risks of the motor car, the motor cycle, the dangers of the Western diet high in saturated fats, to cigarette smoking, or to alcohol, but also to how commercial practices exacerbate these risks.

The growth of a new alcohol epidemiology stressed the relation of alcohol availability, in price, advertising, and age limits in the genesis of alcohol problems. Several broad principles underlie this new alcohol epidemiology. Increases in total alcohol consumption are likely to mean increases in the number of heavy consumers; heavy consumption and damage to health are highly correlated; therefore, preventive programmes must seek to limit increase in general consumption.[13]

The importance of these findings is that they bring into view damages to the community as a whole that arise from changes in the organization of alcohol commerce—production, availability, price, advertising or promotion of alcoholic beverages. Tax policy is a good example. Cook has reviewed the evidence that tax policy is crucial to preventing alcohol related problems like cirrhosis and even drunk driving, and has statistically verified these relationships for the period 1960–1975 in the United States.[14]

Alcohol has long been taxed in most Western democracies, to raise revenue and to discourage consumption. In the United States at the federal level alcohol taxation has been mostly a war tax, and the last major increase was during the Korean War.[15] The tax, levied as an excise or flat tax, was not changed or indexed to inflation. But taxes at all levels of government make up a big part of the price of alcoholic beverages, especially distilled spirits. Because so much of the total price is a fixed and unchanging factor, alcohol prices do not rise as rapidly during inflation as do the prices of goods which are not taxed so highly. Thus, a policy of war taxation, imposed by public officials with few public health motives in mind, resulted in a situation in which the actual price of distilled spirits fell by 48 per cent since 1960. Beer fell in price by 27 per cent.[14]

Tax policy is important not only because of the connection between the price of alcohol, drinking, heavy consumption, and other problems but because tax, along with the number of outlets, the hours of sale, who may sell alcoholic beverages, age restrictions, advertising, and the like are part of the structure of alcohol commerce, and commerce is social in nature, a matter of the common life. But tax policy only partly explains shifts in alcohol consumption. Actually, beer sales increased sharply during the 1970s, while sales of distilled beverages levelled off. The reason for this is that beer is taxed very lightly compared to distilled beverages, and beer is also nationally advertised on American television.

There is little doubt that tax policy and other relaxations on alcohol commerce influence the level of aggregate consumption of alcoholic beverages, including many alcohol-related problems.[14] Even Mill admitted that the market was social. '[T]rade is a social act. Whoever undertakes to sell any description of goods to the public, does what affects the interests of other persons, and of society in general; . . . '.[5] Mill admitted that those who sell alcoholic beverages have an interest in intemperance and therefore restrictions on availability may be justified. 'The interest, however, of these dealers in promoting intemperance is a real evil, and justifies the State in imposing restrictions and requiring guarantees which but for that justification would be infringements of real liberty.' Yet he goes on to rule out taxes for discouraging intemperance as restrictions aimed at the drinker and not at the seller.

But price is little different from restricting the numbers of public houses or supermarkets in a district; both affect availability, the one economic, the other social. And it is this organization of alcohol commerce that is central to any scheme of balancing the community's interest in temperance with the individual's interest in spending his money how he chooses.

Mill argued that only the individual can know his own particular good: 'He is the person most interested in his own wellbeing: the interest which any other person, except in cases of strong personal attachment, can have in it, is trifling, . . . '.[5] But this is precisely the wrong point. Public health paternalism in regulating alcohol commerce seeks to protect the common good, not the good of any particular person. As Richard Flathman notes, modern governments rarely can be paternalistic in the strict sense of promoting the good of particular persons.[16] The liberalization of availability of alcoholic beverages affects the broad drinking public. Historically, government has sought to regulate trade when it affects an important community interest.

TWO CHEERS FOR PATERNALISM

Public health paternalism provides some surprising dividends beyond regulating alcohol commerce and improving the public's health. Strengthening the public health is not only a matter of improving aggregate welfare, it is also encouraging the citizen to share in a group scheme to promote a wider welfare, of which his own welfare is only a part. Seat-belt legislation or signs on the beach restricting swimming when a lifeguard is not present, restrict my liberty for my own good, but only as I am a member of the public and for the general or the common good. From the private viewpoint, the motto for such paternalistic legislation employing the group principle might be, 'The lives we save together might include my own'.

Thus, public health paternalism encourages concern for the wider good, for cooperation, and group solidarity in solving problems. These are community virtues which are needed alongside of the individual virtues of self-reliance and autonomy. National pension schemes may be narrowly paternalistic, but more importantly they encourage group cooperation for the good of everyone alike, stimulating group solidarity. While policies to raise the price of alcohol may seem considerably less concerned with group solidarity than government pension schemes, we should not ignore the possibility that paternalism in life-style areas also advances group values and group approaches to solving problems.

This is speculation, but public health paternalism may also help stimulate individual responsibility, at least up to a point. There is often the view that coercion and individual responsibility operate in a zero-sum manner — seat-belt legislation may cause individuals to take less heed for their own safety on the highway. But it may work the other way around. Fluoridation programmes may help stimulate personal dental hygiene, and government pension schemes may establish a secure minimum around which individuals take voluntary actions to purchase annuities. Similarly, and within limits, community restrictions on drinking and smoking may provide a climate that encourages more individual responsibility regarding drinking or smoking, independently of the direct coercive effect on individuals. Indeed, this might be a main way in which many life-style limitations work.

Another way in which public health paternalism may help strengthen a sense of group as well as individual welfare is through enlarging the sense that the standards behind regulating commerce and life-style choices are based on group norms rather than individual ones. For example, alcohol consumption in most societies for most individuals is far lower than the amount which might be safe for them as private citizens. As a rough yardstick, 'safe drinking' from the individual standpoint is one and a half ounces of absolute alcohol daily, or the equivalent of three glasses of beer. But in the United States, which stands roughly at the mid-point among Western nations in total alcohol consumption, probably less than 15 to 20 per cent of the population drinks that much.[17] Community standards are therefore based on solidarity of interest, meant to reduce the number who suffer alcohol problems. Similarly, seat-belt legislation seeks a group level of safety that individuals acting alone find hard to choose.

How do we keep public health paternalism from going too far and threatening individual autonomy? Do we go from regulating alcohol and the promotion of cigarettes to forbidding rock-climbing? The short answer is no. Public health paternalism focusses on the market place and on those areas where private interests can exploit the public interest. This would include limiting commercial corporations who have a stake in low levels of safety and in risk-taking, to also limiting medical practice to protect the common interest in rationing medical care and in controlling medical expenditure. Public health paternalism mixes controls on providers or producers and consumers and does not seem too intrusive. However, requiring each citizen to jog three miles a day, or to maintain an optimum body weight would bring the state far too close to the individual and would threaten personal autonomy. Commercial regulations and regulating public space operate generally and at a distance, not singling out one particular individual or another for moral improvement. Perhaps the key limit to the balance principle is the presumption it usually carries for individual liberty. Liberty is to be preferred unless regulation guarantees a significant gain to the community. The restrictions sought should also be least restrictive measures available consistent with the ends to be achieved. And the burden of proof is on those who desire the restriction of liberty to demonstrate community benefits.

THREATENING INDIVIDUAL INTERESTS

Antipaternalism may actually increase rather than reduce threats to individual interests. It does this in three separate areas: by focussing on blame, by putting undue stress on children and young people otherwise not of legal age, and by raising the risk of prohibition. Policies which balance community and individual interest actually do a better job of protecting individual interests overall by spreading responsibility for prevention more equitably among the affected interests.

Drunk driving has been the main exception to governments' lack of interest in alcohol policy. In the United States, this issue has led the way for increased national and local attention to alcohol policy. The group responsible is Mothers Against Drunk Drivers (recently renamed Mothers Against Drunk Driving), or MADD which was founded by the charismatic mother of a young girl who was killed by a drunk driver.

Solving social problems by punishing wrongs or crimes is a principal method of those forms of antipaternalism rooted in a strong political individualism. As Mill put it, 'The preventive function of government . . . is far more liable to be abused, to the prejudice of liberty, than the punitory function'.[5] The primary motive behind drunk-driving campaigns is to punish drunk driving as a way of symbolizing the community's repugnance for the practice, and secondly, to deter drunk driving by inflicting stiffer penalties and instituting more effective detection methods. These are legitimate and even important governmental interests.

But increasing the legal penalties and certainty of punishment for drunk driving, taken by itself, is not likely to have permanent and long-term results in reducing this problem. The main reason is the difficulty for police forces in detecting drinking and driving. In the United States the risks of detection in most areas is one in 2000.[18] In England the estimate, even during intense enforcement, is only one in 1000.[18] As Lawrence Ross has noted, campaigns against drinking and driving probably have their effect because they alter the subjective assessment by citizens of the risks of detection.[19] Once the initial wave of publicity passes, the public learns that risk of detection has not increased appreciably, and the previous levels of drunk driving are re-established.

The main problem is that many Western societies have made alcohol so widely available and convenient to the car as to actually constitute a licence to drink and drive. In most Western countries, beer is widely available in most retail establishments, with few government personnel to detect sales to intoxicated or under age people. In many states in the United States it is permissible to drink and drive—only *drunk* driving is forbidden. Western societies have put heavy reliance on detection of drunk driving by the police, with the result that the practice of police stopping drivers randomly to administer sobriety tests is on the increase. What starts out as antipaternalism and legal sanctions winds up as a very serious increase in the level of law enforcement in democratic societies.

Another paradoxical outcome of political individualism is the unusual emphasis given to control and protection of young persons. As Mill argued, the restrictions on limiting society's and the government's power over the adult's private conduct do not apply to young people: 'Society has . . . absolute power over [children and youth] during all the early portion of their existence: it has . . . the whole period of childhood and nonage in which to try whether it could make them capable of rational conduct in life'.[5] Political individualism puts so much stress on leaving the adult free to choose his own ends that, almost of necessity, the young bear the brunt of social control. Defining the community's interest in alcohol policy as principally that of regulating the behaviour of the young can make them the scapegoat for society's policies. Nils Christie has warned that increased governmental interest in alcohol policy is likely to take the form of extending 'childhood' for longer and longer periods to legitimize the supervision by the state.[2] Certainly, the recent experience in the United States, with the federal government's endorsement of a uniform national legal drinking age of 21 years, is partial evidence that this is occurring.

The point is not to ignore the young or punishment for drunk drivers but to balance restrictions and legislation aimed at these groups with broader controls on alcohol commerce that affect the entire population. As Michael Grossman argues, a slight increase in the tax on beer might save as many lives as a one year increase in the age limit for drinking.[20] The other advantage of this policy is that it would also help prevent problems among those who are older as well, and would also make the young feel less singled out. Policies against drunk driving—whether aimed at the young or not—might also include limitation on the availability of alcohol in the retail distribution system, an increase in the level of surveillance of that system by state liquor licence personnel, or an increase in the price of alcoholic beverages, especially beer. Better yet, we could do all three things at once. The growing application of civil liability for retail operators who serve under age or drunk patrons or both is also likely to help reduce the problem, and to shift attention away from the criminal justice system.

There is yet another danger to individual interests from the undue focus on blame in many kinds of antipaternalism. This is the danger of what has come to be called 'victim blaming'[21] which is discussed more fully in Chapter 9. Victim blaming begins by noting that smoking and alcohol abuse add significant social costs to society, especially by lost productivity and increased medical and insurance costs. The next step is to argue that these groups should be held accountable for these costs to the others in society. As one American critic has argued, '[O]ne man's freedom in health is another man's shackle in taxes and insurance premiums'.[22] But where does this principle of individual responsibility to the larger society end? Are the obese, those with large families, those who fail to exercise also to be similarly burdened? Thus, it is a short step from a position of individual autonomy to a position of social responsibility to the larger society, from a position of individual autonomy to social stigmatization.

This position of making the risk-taker pay his own way ignores the extent to which drinking and smoking as actions are a complex bundle of voluntary and involuntary features, structural as well as individual causal relationships. While we should not ignore the role of choice, alcohol and cigarettes are also powerfully addictive and heavily promoted by commercial interests. The community position would spread the responsibility more broadly, seeing these problems as *both* community and individual problems, using prevention rather than blame and measures aimed at all who smoke or drink, as well as the industries.

Finally, there is the paradox of prohibition itself. It is striking that the country that experienced the longest period of national prohibition, the United States, is the democracy that comes nearer to a public philosophy of political individualism. Prohibition came to the United States for many complex reasons. One of the reasons is surely that, when problems such as alcohol abuse become so severe that society has to take action, the militant antipaternalist is forced either to revise his antipaternalism or to escalate seriously the threat that alcohol itself poses to the individual. This is what seems to have happened with the shift from the early temperance drives which were voluntary in character, and which met with limited success. Prohibition came next, and it came in significant part because the philosophy of political individualism offered no middle ground for balancing regulation of alcohol use with its continued commercial availability. Antipaternalist philosophies nearly always contain room for substances or conditions which are so inherently dangerous that extreme government regulation and even prohibition is justified. When a balancing approach is not popularly embraced or understood, there is a strong temptation to take a newly problematic set of conditions (the rise of the saloon in the nineteenth century) and a substance (alcohol) and reclassify it in the same group that today is reserved for drugs like heroin. Room for compromise and balance is thus lost, because why should a dangerous drug be allowed in the stream of commerce? This experience might serve as a cautionary tale for commercial interests who defend their interests in the name of political individualism.

So, two cheers for paternalism—public health paternalism. Public health paternalism permits a sharing of responsibility for controlling the impulses of one's life, and for strengthening those motives of cooperation and trust that are the cornerstone of the community.[23] As with everything else, this principle has its dangers, but societies which ignore the needs of community and mutual dependency are deeply unwise, encouraging the very threats to private interests that they so noisily and blindly seek to protect.

REFERENCES

1. Lukes, S. *Individualism*. New York: Harper and Row, 1973: 79–87.
2. Christie, N. Foreword. **In**: Markela, K., Room, R., Single, E., Sulkunen, P. and Walsh, B. *Alcohol, Society, and the State. A Comparative Study of Alcohol Control*. Toronto: Addiction Research Foundation, 1981: xiv.
3. Barry, B. *The Liberal Theory of Justice*. Oxford: Clarendon, 1973.
4. Thompson, I. E. The ethical debate. **In**: Grant, M., Ritson, B. *Alcohol—the Prevention Debate*. London: Croom Helm, 1983: 171–179.
5. Mill, J. S. On liberty. **In**: Cohen, M. (ed). *The Philosophy of John Stuart Mill*. New York: Modern Library, 1961: 185–319.
6. Schelling, T. *Micromotives and Macrobehavior*. New York: Norton, 1978.
7. Hirsch, F. *Social Limits to Growth*. Cambridge: Harvard, 1978.
8. Peters, R. M. Jr. *The Massachusetts Constitution of 1780—a Social Compact*. Amherst, Massachusetts: University of Massachusetts Press, 1978.
9. Levy, L. *The Law of the Commonwealth and Chief Justice Shaw*. Cambridge: Harvard University Press, 1957.
10. *Mugler versus Kansas*. 123 US, 1887.
11. Makela, K., Room, R., Single, E., Sulkunen, P. and Walsh, B. *Alcohol, Society, and the State. A Comparative Study of Alcohol Control*. Toronto: Addiction Research Foundation, 1981.
12. Terris, M. The changing relationships of epidemiology and society: the Robert Cruikshank lecture. *J Pub Hlth Policy* 1985; **6**: 15–36.

13. Schmidt, W. and Popham, R. Discussion of paper by Parker and Harman. **In**: Harford, T. C., Parker, D. A. and Light, L. *Normative Approaches to the Prevention of Alcohol Abuse and Alcoholism*. Research Monograph No. 3. National Institute on Alcohol Abuse and Alcoholism. Department of Health and Human Services. Washington, DC: United States Government Printing Office, 1980.
14. Cook, P. J. The effect of liquor taxes on drinking, cirrhosis, and auto accidents. **In**: Moore, M. and Gerstein, D. (eds). *Alcohol and Public Policy: Beyond the Shadow of Prohibition*. Washington, DC: National Academy Press, 1981.
15. Mosher, J. and Beauchamp, D. Justifying alcohol taxes to public officials. *J Pub Hlth Policy* 1983; **4**: 422–439.
16. Flathman, R. *The public interest; an essay concerning the normative discourse of politics*. New York: Wiley, 1966.
17. Beauchamp, D. *Beyond Alcoholism: Alcohol and Public Health Policy*. Philadelphia: Temple University Press, 1980.
18. Reed, D. S. Reducing the costs of drinking and driving. **In**: Moore, M. and Gerstein D. *Alcohol and Public Policy: Beyond the Shadow of Prohibition*. Washington, DC: National Academy Press, 1981: 336–387.
19. Ross, H. L. Law, science, and accidents: the British road safety act of 1967. *J Legal Stud* 1973; **2**: 1–78.
20. Grossman, M., Coate, D. and Arluck, G. Price sensitivity of alcoholic beverages in the US. Paper presented at the Conference on Control Issues in Alcohol Abuse Prevention: Impacting Communities. South Carolina Commission on Alcohol and Drug Abuse, Charleston, SC, October 7–10, 1984.
21. Ryan, W. *Blaming the Victim*. Vintage: New York, 1976.
22. Knowles, J. H. The responsibility of the individual. **In**: Knowles, J. H. (ed). *Doing Better and Feeling Worse*. New York: Norton, 1977.
23. Slater, P. *The Pursuit of Loneliness*. Boston: Beacon, 1970.

Ethical Dilemmas in Health Promotion
Edited by S. Doxiadis

CHAPTER 8

Health Legislation, Prevention and Ethics

GENEVIEVE PINET

SUMMARY

The observed progress in the introduction of health legislation in Western industrial societies reflects a generally increasing concern about health issues. Traditionally legislation has dealt with the needs of curative medicine and in certain areas of prevention, notably in the control of infectious disease and in the care of certain vulnerable groups in society. Present trends, however, have resulted from enlarged concepts of health, new definitions of prevention and changing perspectives about the role of legislation in the promotion of health. Law is seen as an instrument which can have an influence in the primary, secondary and tertiary prevention of disease, and in the promotion of health generally, whether by influencing life-styles or counteracting adverse environments. Notwithstanding these tendencies, the laws are introduced against a background of intense debate, reflecting conflicts in interests, policies and principles. In addition the increasing rate of technical and scientific advance in the medical sciences raises important debates about ethical standards in society. The chapter is divided broadly into three parts, the first of which draws attention to the increasing role of legislation in the health field. The next section addresses questions and conflicts raised by government intervention, and discusses the practical and ethical problems of attempting to use legislation for the prevention of disease—efforts to control the environment and to change life-styles are taken as examples. The last part discusses the contribution of health legislation in supporting preventive action applied to the whole range of comprehensive care—health protection, diagnosis, treatment and rehabilitation and health promotion—taking into account the ethical issues inherent in this approach.

TRENDS IN HEALTH LEGISLATION

The protection of health through legal measures has been the concern of national and international interests especially since this second half of the

20th century and after the creation of the United Nations with its specialized agencies, in particular the World Health Organization (WHO).

Since then the emphasis placed on the development of human rights has been matched simultaneously by the necessity to recognize the right to health. In this respect one may refer to the preamble of the Constitution of the WHO of 1946: 'The enjoyment of the highest attainable standard of health is one of the fundamental rights of every human being without distinction of race, religion, political belief, economic or social condition'. Within the modern concept of the right to health we can see three elements—the right to health within its individual, community and international dimensions; the right to 'the highest attainable standard of health' as a fundamental human right; the right to self-determination and to participate in the achievements of society.

In this context, an increasing number of governments have stressed in their national legislation or in their constitution or in both 'the right to health care' as a fundamental principle for activities in the health field. Obviously, the right to health care is limited in practice by the degree to which resources are available. If up to now it was essentially a question of the right to health, with all that this supposes, there is now a need to go further and to establish the rights of patients. In several countries there is evidence of public demand that the rights of the patients be clearly established—for instance, the right to information, to protection of privacy, to freedom of choice, to refusal of treatment. Thus we witness an increasing development of legislation in support of patients' rights, both at national and international levels where charters of patients' rights are proposed. Legislation supports also the emergence of new patients' rights. There is, furthermore, a considerable amount of legislation to guarantee the rights of special groups of patients, such as the disabled, mental patients, patients in hospitals. Ethical codes have kept an importance but there is a clear trend to have what were once doctors' duties reformulated as legal rights of patients.

PROBLEMS OF GOVERNMENT INTERVENTION

The traditional role of law, to formulate rights and duties, to express policy, to balance the interests of the various sectors of society, to protect individuals and the community, to set up norms and standards, extends itself to the field of health.

Health legislation is both an expression of a stated health policy and an instrument by which governments seek to strengthen their health activities. Decision-making, the crucial act of politics, may remain dormant if not backed up by legislation. Legislation further provides the managerial and administrative basis for the development of health systems. Legislation intervenes to balance public interest and rights of the individual in the protection of health. Health legislation is also instrumental in settling conflicts of interest between various groups of our industrialized society whose activities have important repercussions on the health and wellbeing of populations.

The increasing importance of health in society leads to an increasing intervention of the legislator in health affairs. To give effect to a particular health policy, a government can use different approaches, either direct or indirect, by encouragement or subsidy of third parties. One of the recent approaches is found in the entry of the legislator into the field of health promotion and life-style, where the interesting combination of educative, compulsory and incentive measures constitutes an original strategy—an example of this is legislation on the compulsory wearing of seat-belts in cars. Legislation that provides incentives for healthy behaviour, for example through tax benefits or by influencing the way in which insurance rates are structured, is a kind of persuasive role much milder than coercion. Legislation may support the government policy of education of the population and community participation. The state can have an educational role, and without infringing individual freedom in any way, can engage in a campaign of public education that relies on the judgment of individuals, to make voluntary changes on how they live. A government could also undertake to support public health activities run by likeminded independent private forces and non-governmental bodies—for example, health insurance companies and other institutions, professional and consumers' associations.

But the role of the state in public health should not be overstated, nor should the difficulties be underplayed. In many countries, for example, governments are reluctant to take appropriate measures to tackle the problems of alcohol abuse because those governments are primarily interested in the production, distribution and consumption of alcohol. This problem is dealt with very fully in Chapter 7. Another examples lies in the field of health education to encourage the public to lead healthier lives. We may advise people to eat brown bread and bran and to take exercise. But in doing so we should take into account such factors as higher price of brown bread and its lower availability, or the difficulties faced by the single person living in a high-rise apartment block. We educate for healthier life-styles but do not facilitate them. And government with its complex responsibilities and concerns with taxation, importation, distribution and so forth, quite often resists this particular role.

When government does act, resistance may well come from those for whose benefit the preventive measures are being taken. There is a great deal to be said for allowing the value of particular measures to be understood by the population before these measures are imposed by the State. Greater reliance by governments on the public conscience or public opinion might improve considerably eventual acceptance of a particular law. In fact, health professionals and politicians have realized, especially in the industrialized countries, that further progress in improving community health will have to come about through alterations in habits. This involves giving encouragement to individuals and groups to adopt healthy life-styles and health legislation can serve as an indirect approach for this purpose.

This brings us to another point of interest, the choice of legal methods. The legal tool can adapt itself to various purposes in the preventive field—for instance: *comprehensive or categorical legislation* of which the environmental sector provides many examples; *direct or indirect legislation* to influence individual behaviour; *regulatory legislation* which is much used in food control for security and quality purposes; *enabling legislation* to provide financial support for sports facilities such as swimming pools or bicycle paths; *referendum to enact legislation* in the context of a public issue such as fluoridation of the public water supply.

Limitations to Legislation

Reasons for the intervention of the legislator, particularly because of the growing awareness of the importance of health in our society, can be understood quite readily. The limitations to such intervention are less obvious. From society's point of view there are various commonly accepted principles for public interference with individual autonomy—hazards to others or society as a whole, as in the case of preventing the threat of communicable diseases, or to guarantee public order threatened by mentally disordered patients; nature of constraint, for instance the obligation to wear seat-belts is felt to be different from that of being obliged to drink fluoridated water; degree of dangerousness in the invasion of human physical and mental integrity potentially involved in some types of clinical research.

Parallel to these two developments—the increasing concern of the society for its health and the increasing intervention of the health-legislator—one can also observe the increasing role of the consumers in society, particularly in the recognition of the serious impact of psycho-social factors on health. The needs of consumers, expressed or felt, are being backed up by consumers' associations and pressure groups which have an influence on the passing of legislation on specific subjects. The question arises of determining how the participation of the consumers of health care can be achieved in the formulation of health policy and decision-making. The ways of effecting consumer involvement in government intervention are very varied. However, participation of the consumer in health issues where professionals predominate will not be realized without the support of legislation.

Questions are raised by government intervention through legislation in the field of prevention and related ethical issues. Governments have to act in a vast and complex field of sensitive issues, involving social, economic, technical and ethical which interact and give rise to conflicts of interest, principles and policies. Final decisions on imposing specific measures are often difficult to reach, especially when interests conflict. This can be illustrated by two examples, one concerning the environment and the second relating to life-style.

During the last decade, the prevention of environmental pollution has provided many examples of such conflicts. The intervention of government seemed appropriate in many situations. However, a serious problem cropped up in the early 1980s as a result of the 'acid rain' threat. While this was not a new problem, it had acquired greater dimensions and alarming proportions. Acid rain is found to be responsible for the progressive and continuously increasing deterioration of forests in several European countries. It also harms the biological life of lakes, not to mention the damage caused to ancient monuments. The possible permanent detrimental effects on the ecological balance and on the health of populations causes serious concern to governments and people. The technological solutions to prevent such pollution seem to be available. Where, then, is the issue? The main atmospheric polluters responsible for acid rain are heavy industry, factories and plants using coal, and motor vehicles. The costs or sacrifices of implementing anti-pollution measures prove to be so high that they would threaten the life of the factories, especially when they already find themselves under threat because of financial difficulties. Closing a factory means loss of production and increased unemployment, and this presents the dilemma for a government. With regard to motor vehicles, it is also possible to reduce the pollution resulting from the fuel-combustion to an acceptable level by the use of catalytic mufflers. But this remains a costly proposition for the competitively minded car industry which would not comply unless forced by law. It also implies using lead-free petrol, a switch in production that some European governments are not yet ready to make. Here then is another dilemma for government—a thriving economy versus protected environment. Unfortunately, the member states of the European Economic Communities have difficulty in agreeing to the rapid introduction of catalytic mufflers and the compromise solution that European countries have recently adopted will postpone considerably the measures which are necessary today. If pollution by sulphur dioxide continues, the ecological damage progresses, and these ethical problems remain unsolved, what kind of a legacy will be left to the next generation?

The second example of conflict in legislation concerns its use to promote healthy life-styles. The crucial debate centres on the argument that since life-style is a matter for the individual, the legitimacy of governmental action is questionable and could be considered as interference with people's freedom of action and choice. The conflict here is between protecting public health and ensuring individual liberty. Because freedom in our society is highly valued, any limitation imposed upon it must be justified. Public opinion is very sensitive on matters of encroachment of individual rights. The central ethical problem faced by health decision-makers is that of serving the interest of the community while simultaneously respecting their rights as individuals and preserving their freedom.

So what are the limits on a government's regulatory powers in the light of such dilemmas? In this context several questions recur: how can the value of individual freedom and common good in the field of health be reconciled?; when should the rights of society take precedence over the rights of an individual?; how much can the State interfere with the private behaviour of citizens, even in their best interest, and what is the point beyond which government regulation becomes government intrusion?; what type of legal measures are acceptable and effective in motivating individuals to change their behaviour?; what tactics of implementation of legislation are useful?

Answers to these questions are elusive but the questions themselves are useful in examining attempts to strike the right balance between the goal of successfully changing behaviour related to health and the threshold of acceptance of government interference.

There is, however, one issue in which a consensus can be found—the necessity to obtain the acceptance of the public to the measure proposed. Little will be achieved in trying to induce behavioural changes through legal measures if public opinion has not been properly prepared. A law, even the soundest one, that does not have public support, cannot be implemented.

After these considerations on health, legislation and ethics and related issues on their interface, I should like to add two general remarks, one addressed primarily to the lawyers, the other to the physicians, the two main professional agents involved in the subject.

In reading the work of lawyers in this field, they seem sometimes ill at ease because they are accustomed to relying on clear-cut definitions and well-defined concepts. They tend to resent having to face several differing definitions which may seem too vague to the legal mind. What confounds them also is that when they feel they finally reach the limits of the concept of health, they are then confronted by efforts to enlarge it by including new health-related sectors. Some new health-related sectors have sometimes vague if not controversial definitions—the boundaries of environmental health, for example, remain an issue. And it is true also that defining prevention in the health field is complicated by the evolution of the concept of health. However, it is certainly a good thing to be able to enlarge the concept of health and to find new approaches, taking advantage of the benefits produced by the unprecedented progress of medicine and public health during the last decade.

With regard to the medical profession also there is no unanimity on the meaning of prevention. Differing definitions abound and vary considerably on whether the term is taken in a broad or a restricted sense. Some clinicians in particular in private practice or hospitals have been so overly concerned with the curative effect of medicine and surgery, that they have overlooked their preventive aspects. They are disease rather than health-orientated and still firmly believe that the medical activities and health policy should be centred around curative medicine and the care of sick people in contrast to preventive services for healthy persons. There remains, therefore, a tendency to leave only a secondary role for the preventive aspects of medicine. In this respect you may have noticed that in the title of this paper, I have chosen the word prevention rather than preventive medicine. The choice is deliberate because modern prevention in the health field goes far beyond the realm of the clinical medical prevention. The medical act, while essential, is only one of many in the whole picture of community health action. Prevention and comprehensive community health involve most of the important sectors of health activities today.

LEGISLATION AND TOTAL HEALTH CARE

In the third part of the chapter, I will use a simplified definition of prevention in the health field, a definition of practical interest and one that serves our purpose—'Prevention is not only the act of taking a series of measures designed to avoid the occurrence, as well as the progression of disease and permanent disability, but also the timely application of all means of promoting the health of the individuals and the community as a whole'. In this third part, therefore, the approach to prevention is based on the now classical World Health Organization concept, in line with the extension of the scope of prevention, considering three levels of application of preventive measures—primary, secondary, and tertiary. My intention is to illustrate the contribution health legislation could make on these different aspects of prevention applied to the whole range of comprehensive care, usually described under the four following categories of service—health protection, health recovery through diagnosis and treatment, rehabilitation, and health promotion.

Primary Prevention by Health Protection

The main objective of health protection—sometimes called health maintenance—is to keep people healthy through avoiding the occurrence of illness and accidents by working on their causes and risk factors in a given community. Health protection has been mentioned first because it is the field of original prevention, the traditional preventive medicine, renamed as primary prevention. This is prevention in its conventional meaning which comprises measures applicable to a particular disease or type of accident in order to intercept their causes or avoid the exposure to risks even before they involve man. It is prevention at its best.

Much has already been accomplished in specific protection against communicable diseases in particular. The notification of certain types of diseases and the success of powerful tools like vaccination were ensured by an effective series of compulsory measures through the intervention of law. It is also without doubt the most convincing example of the synergy between law and prevention, without which the most spectacular achievement recently recorded, the eradication of smallpox, would have been impossible. We can speculate too on the state of the health of the world population deprived of the World Health

Organization's International Health regulations. Without strictly enforced preventive international sanitary regulations where would we be in public health today in terms of pandemics, given the enormous and ever-increasing socio-economic phenomenon of movements of populations through tourism and business on a global scale?

In connection with infections and intoxications, we can move on to those transmitted by food and enter upon the wide and topical subject of the security and quality of food products. This provides an excellent example of the combined action of primary prevention and legislation at the national level, with international repercussions because of the increasing growth of tourism and of intercountry trade of food products. All European countries have now passed appropriate legislation to ensure the necessary control for the safety and quality of food products, usually through a long process started, in some cases, at the end of the last century.

Control of the spread of communicable diseases and the safety of food are two instances where legal measures taken by the State have been an efficient means of protecting the health of the public and lends support to the concept of some coercion in the field of prevention. On a smaller scale, in the framework of collective action with acceptance from a majority of the population are the specific protective measures aimed at the prevention of nutritional disorders, such as goitre or dental caries through regulations on iodization of salt or fluoridation of drinking water respectively.

Legislation has long provided support for various preventive programmes on certain community groups, for instance the classical maternal and child health examinations and later on the school health examinations, when, in both occasions, compulsory immunization in particular have to be initiated or updated.

Another important type of preventive action is found in the field of occupational health in which specific protective measures against occupational hazards have been gradually built up over a long period of time and this area is discussed more fully in Chapter 11. More recently, preventive measures were enacted for specific protection of workers and the working environment against the growing toxic hazards of certain rapidly developing industries.

Finally, more recent use of legislation at the primary level of prevention is found in programmes for road traffic accident prevention: regulating speed limits, prohibiting children from riding in the front seat, enforcing the wearing of seat-belts in motor cars, imposing helmets for motor cyclists and so on. Statistics definitely show that these very straightforward coercive measures help to reduce the major problem of road accident epidemics. Although some countries have been much opposed to some of these measures, in such cases the limitation of personal freedom is minimal compared with the gains obtained.

Secondary Prevention by Diagnosis and Treatment

If the chance offered by primary prevention has been missed, and the occurrence of illness or accident could not be avoided, we must appeal to the curative arm to restore health. Here secondary prevention may also be accomplished through early diagnosis and prompt treatment. The plan is to intervene as soon as possible to arrest at the earliest stage or to retard the progress of the existing disease, to shorten its duration, to reduce its consequences, and particularly to avoid complications and sequelae. In other words, the preventive framework called secondary prevention may prevent acute illness from becoming chronic disability.

Secondary prevention can be done through early detection, either by the attending physician during a consultation not necessarily for the original reason, or through a social scheme of selective screening. For example, specific screening measures for diabetes, hypertension, phenylketonuria, are of proven value, although the efficacy of a global screening programme remains doubtful. Thus public health laws could favour the potential benefits to be derived by sound specific preventive measures directed towards high risk and vulnerable groups. In terms of treatment, a situation can arise in which legal action is used to prevent spread to others if the disease is a communicable one—for instance, sexually transmitted diseases, tuberculosis and other infectious diseases.

In our modern industrialized countries, however, infectious diseases are tending to disappear, and we are now faced with the problem of degenerative disease, the two main preoccupying ones being cancer and cardio-cerebro-vascular diseases. Their control by early detection of the latent disease in high-risk groups, that is to say through screening and treatment of the first symptoms is already proving to be very rewarding. This underlines the usefulness of public health programmes of secondary prevention backed by legislation.

Tertiary Prevention by Rehabilitation

We are now moving towards the third phase of comprehensive care, the field of rehabilitation. This is a step further than stabilizing or stopping the disease or accident process. It is a set of measures to avoid further deterioration, to escape in particular the establishment of an irreversible disability. It is, above all, to prevent a permanent handicap. The measures taken to that effect after treatment has been applied, are known as tertiary prevention. The main objective of tertiary prevention through rehabilitative measures is to return the affected individual to a normal place in society and allow maximum use of his or her remaining capacities.

The success of rehabilitation depends upon the provision of work therapy in hospital, of community facilities for vocational training, of good referral services to the proper institution. It entails, among other things, selective placement techniques, and education of both public and industry in the value and employability of the rehabilitated.

Rehabilitation has physical, psychological, vocational and economic components which have many implications in the socio-medical field. And a complex and comprehensive rehabilitation programme can only exist with the strong support of various appropriate legislative measures.

The possibilities offered by modern rehabilitation call for a heavy contribution by the medical and social services—for example, the cost of corrective surgery, the provision of prostheses, rehabilitative measures, and training of highly specialized personnel. These services are costly not only in terms of money but also of time and labour. Cost is the greatest deterrent to the rapid extension of rehabilitative services. Legislation has to be introduced to ensure equity in the allocation of financial resources and as well in access to rehabilitation facilities. In industrialized countries the legislative tool is usually well developed either as specific legislation, or as legislation integrated to the one for medical care. While legislation in most European countries includes provisions for disabled persons, more attention should be paid to promoting legislation on preventing disability.

Third level prevention aims at preventing disabilities from developing into handicap—that is, consequences which limit or prevent the fulfilment of the individual's normal role in society. The measures required usually correspond to rehabilitation of the disabled. It is, however, important to stress the preventive component of such action because it places some emphasis on measures, going far beyond medical action, such as barrier-free design of new public buildings and homes which will prevent many disabled with locomotor problems from becoming mobility handicapped. Special attention should also be paid to the abolition of existing architectural barriers, because they still prevent many disabled people from becoming socially integrated. Appropriate legislation may be required to encourage the application of barrier-free design.

Rehabilitation is a preventive and service programme for all types and ages of patients and people. The elderly are a particularly interesting group for two reasons. Firstly, the proportion of people over the age of 60 years will increase in the next 20 years in European countries and it is in the 80–85 year age-group that the rate of increase will be the highest. Secondly, the risk of suffering from handicap increases with age. Thus, the increasing proportion of older people together with the increasing risk of disability can only magnify the problem of rehabilitation. Unless decisive action is taken now, there is an indication that the number of disabled people could double by the end of the century. Thus there is great interest in legal initiatives by governments in taking appropriate measures to support tertiary prevention aimed particularly at avoiding the loss of independence. As a consequence, tertiary prevention will also be prevention against dependence upon the family or the community. Rehabilitative measures offer the opportunity not only of alleviating suffering, but also of reducing the burden upon society to support helplessly disabled and psychologically maladjusted patients, a remarkable humanitarian goal and a challenging social issue.

Health Promotion

Within the framework of the transition from the state of health to the state of disease we have already considered three sequential aspects of comprehensive care and their corresponding levels of prevention. But there is nowadays increasing insistence on preventive measures taking place at an earlier level, before health protection. This is known as health promotion, and here the health concept becomes more dynamic. The notion of wellbeing is transcended by the notion of quality of life. It is an evolving concept that encompasses fostering life-styles and environmental factors conducive to health. This is not surprising when we consider that many of our present illnesses, so-called diseases of modern civilization, have a mainly environmental and behavioural origin.

Health promotion measures are an extension of primary prevention because they depend on taking action against causal factors detrimental to health and that in fact health promotion and health protection overlap to a certain extent when put into practice.

The environment is one of the most fertile areas for health promotion. In this context, it implies measures to improve living conditions and the ecological factors which influence the development of human and social progress. These include the provision of suitable housing, the monitoring of safe water and food quality, adequate recreational and sport facilities, green spaces, efficient transport systems and attention to the environmental aspects of accident prevention. The problems encountered are usually solved by conventional measures in community health taken at the local or regional level. Health authorities, for example, watch that requirements stipulated by sanitary rules and regulations and compliance with environmental standards have been fulfilled.

In environmental terms, health promotion also implies guarding against dangers to health caused by pollution from physical or chemical sources, radioactivity, or noise. This means in particular, control of industrial production. The management of man's environment is a field in which government action by means of legislation is particularly appropriate and it can be decided upon in a relatively centralized manner. People and communities in fact have limited or indeed no influence on such risks and must rely on the legislator to protect them. There is now another, perhaps more compelling, motivation for the legislator—the necessity to deal with long-range problems. If it is urgent to succeed in protecting the present generation from the short-range damage to the quality of our lives and our environment, it is practically and morally important to protect future generations from the long-term effects of certain nuisances and pollutants affecting the planet and its atmosphere. The storage of radioactive waste and as already mentioned, the problems of acid rain are two such examples. Here the issue of implementation is extremely important and the intervention of national and international authorities is needed.

The protection of the environment is a public matter, a matter of state and interstate responsibility, where many interests conflict, and it has to be guaranteed by legislative measures.

In spite of potential difficulties, impressive achievements have been recorded in many sectors of pollution control. The constant debate about environment has raised a collective consciousness which greatly facilitates the use of law to intervene efficiently. Particularly worthy of mention are the gratifying results now obtained in the substantial reduction and efficient monitoring of numerous aspects of air and water pollution in many European industrialized countries. The encouraging progress that has been made in dealing with environmental health problems are beyond a doubt the result of the environmental health legislation enacted and implemented during the last decade. This reflects the importance of law as a tool in the quest for better environment and improved public health. But it is also in this area that the most frightening threats to health may occur as we have seen in the huge industrial catastrophes in Seveso, Mexico, Bhopal and more recently in Chernobyl. This is a very cruel way of reminding us of the need to strengthen legislation to grant higher protection for populations living in higher risk industrial areas. Transportation of dangerous goods and international movements of noxious products and wastes with the least hazard is another pressing environmental issue to be regulated by governments. Countries also have to rely on international environmental legislation to protect them.

Health promotion also involves efforts to increase physical, mental and emotional wellbeing. One way to achieve this is by improving individual behaviour which has been labelled life-style choice. In terms of prevention this means avoiding harmful personal habits. Food intake, alcohol consumption, tobacco smoking, physical exercise and so forth are health-related choices. The important point is that the decisions taken are under the control of the individual since he has the capability to take the health risks of his or her choice, sometimes referred to as voluntary health risks.

Voluntary Health Risks

Here we are entering the core of an ethical problem. To what extent should society tolerate those personal health risk choices which appear to have dangerous repercussions upon others? Let us take the example of one such health risk, smoking. Tobacco smoking is one of the greatest current self-inflicted dangers to health and there is no doubt at present of the part played by tobacco in the causation or exacerbation of numerous diseases. But faced with this risk people are not equal—because of specific responses particular to each individual, cardiac, pulmonary, cancer risks are considerable for some and less for others. In terms of prevention it would be interesting to detect the most vulnerable individuals and to compile a risk profile. This might lead to information enabling individuals to be made aware of their specific risks. This preventive approach is complementary to the one which is global and indiscriminate. It is in the general line of the traditional medical approach which tries to be personal and to go beyond collective rules in order to study the situation of each person concerned.

A newly debated problem is that of passive tobacco intoxication which may be defined as the exposure of non-smokers to the combustion of tobacco products in a closed environment. It would seem that the smoking of others can no longer be considered as innocuous. Smoking is far more than a simple nuisance and implies a toxic risk for the environment. Contrary to the case of alcoholic consumption, the non-consumption of tobacco is not sufficient to avoid a risk because of the pollution of the air by smokers, for example, in public and professional premises and private homes. During pregnancy, for example, a mother who smokes subjects her fetus to the negative effects of passive tobacco intoxication. The risk of premature birth, undernutrition of the newborn, and further developmental troubles, are well known as possible consequences.

Equally well known is the indifference of smokers to their surroundings be they public, professional or private. Indeed, the harm from passive smoking raises problems of ethics and individual freedom. In this respect it is important that the public at large be informed as objectively as possible. The legislators should investigate this severe problem because it opens the way to practical conclusions and the adoption of reasonable laws or recommendations which take into account the protection of the individual and in particular the protection of children, without, however, ostracizing the smoker completely.

To approach the problem of voluntary health risks objectively is to raise many an ethical question. Has the individual the right to take voluntary health risks of his or her choice? Do any voluntary health risks in fact exist since we are all very much influenced by our genetic inheritance, educational pattern, social standing, family habits and religious beliefs? Can society intervene only when the individual presents a danger to others, as sometimes in communicable diseases, alcoholism or certain types of mental illnesses? Do we allow a certain degree of paternalism in such situations as sometimes found in the wording of professional codes? Why should society bear the burden of its citizens' taking risks with their own health, particularly when many social security systems are obliged to pay the bill and when the diminishing resources force a selection among the patients or extend the waiting time for the treatment of someone else?

Would it be possible to have legislation that requires separate insurance assessments for voluntary risk-takers in cases where voluntary risks are involved? Such questions are actually being raised in view of the serious situation facing the financing of health services. Because of the lasting economic crisis, most countries are now trying to halt the continued growth of health services expenditure.

The end of this century is likely to be marked by low economic growth or even no growth. It could be unwise to count on appreciable increase in the resources that countries could or would be prepared to devote to health services in the next 15 years.

To a large extent, it will be necessary to correct the shortcomings of health services and meet new needs by making the present systems more efficient, by redistributing the existing resources to make them more cost-effective, by encouraging people to take responsibility for their own health, and by thus reducing the undue burden on services that has resulted from insufficient attention being paid to prevention in the past. A striking example is the enormous costs of curative hospital-based services in traumatology. Traumatic injuries resulting from work, sports, driving, too often result from accidents which could have been avoided by proper preventive action. The economic situation we now face calls for new priorities to be set for appropriate revision of much of the existing health legislation.

Is health now so valued in our society that a prevalent idea of social justice would hold an individual responsible to the community for his or her own health? Some may feel that if we go too far in this direction there is a danger of victimization of the sick by overstressing individual responsibility towards health and governments might also be tempted to abandon some existing preventive health action. By overstressing the health aspects of life-style we could also end up with a kind of medicalization of society which would be almost the reverse of the original intention of the preventive action. Others, however, may feel that, in the realm of illness clearly related to personal behaviour, the community has the right to expect the individual to be responsible for his risk choices which impinge on the health or finances of the society.

These are moral and ethical issues which await society's judgment. How should these ethical health issues be dealt with? First society must make its ethical choice as to the degree of responsibility of the individual and society on this matter. Once a decision has been made, it can be implemented through a combination of educational, incentive and compulsory measures. But these ethical dilemmas require much study and discussion.

CONCLUSION

The unprecedented achievements of research and of progress in biotechnology raise ethical problems which are of great current concern in law, in public health, in government and in society in general. But in closing I would like to emphasize that we have also reached a turning point in prevention which has now become a dynamic and evolutionary process taking advantage of the new possibilities of biotechnology, the tools of modern epidemiology, the input of social sciences, information resources, the techniques of the media and health education, and the possibilities of health legislation, whose resources have not yet been fully used. The following quotation from a statement by Sir George Young, former Minister of Health of the United Kingdom, could not better summarize the task ahead in prevention and its ethical dilemmas: 'The solution of many present health problems will not be found in hospital research laboratories but in our parliaments. Diseases which kill most nowadays are due to our life-style and the reaction against these illnesses is not cure but prevention'.

GENERAL REFERENCES

Beauchamp, D. E. Public Health and Individual Liberty. *Ann Rev Public Health* 1980; 121–36.

Fielding, J. E. Lessons from Health Care Regulation. *Ann Rev Public Health* 1983; 91–130.

WHO. *First International Course on Health Legislation*. Copenhagen: World Health Organization, Regional Office for Europe, 1984.

Kallio, V. *Medical and Social Problems of the Disabled*. Copenhagen: World Health Organization, Regional Office for Europe, 1982.

Leenen, H. J. J., Pinet, G. and Prims, A. V. *Trends in Health Legislation in Europe*. Copenhagen/Paris: WHO/MASSON, 1986.

Ligneau, P. *La prévention Sanitaire en France. Revue de Droit Sanitaire et Sociale*. Paris: Sirey, 1983.

Martin, J. *A propos du rôle de la Législation sanitaire, notamment en rélation avec la prévention*. Copenhagen: World Health Organization, Regional Office for Europe, 1981.

Regional Targets in support of the Regional Strategy for Health for All. Copenhagen: World Health Organization, Regional Office for Europe, 1984.

Veatch, R. M. and Taylor, B. (eds). *Health Promotion! Ethical Considerations in Health Promotion Principles and Clinical Applications*. Norwalk, Connecticut: Appleton Century Crofts, 1982.

Yan Kauer, A. Public and private prevention. *Ann J Public Health* 1983; **73**: 1032–34.

Ethical Dilemmas in Health Promotion
Edited by S. Doxiadis

CHAPTER 9

Value Conflicts in Social Policies for Promoting Health

LEON EISENBERG

SUMMARY

In so far as measures to promote health require changes in behaviour (abandoning old habits and acquiring new ones), they challenge implicit value preferences. Since individuals differ in the values they assign to future health as opposed to present comforts, conflict is inevitable when such measures become government policy urged or enforced on all citizens. Yet the health of the population is necessarily a central concern for all governments, with its ramifications extending from matters of social justice to decisions on the allocation of tax funds. In this chapter I will attempt to illuminate these issues by comparing the responsibility of the individual for his or her own health with the responsibility of society for the health of all of its members, using as my main example the family planning policy of the People's Republic of China.

LEVELS OF DISEASE PREVENTION IN PUBLIC HEALTH

Public health terminology distinguishes among three levels of disease prevention. Primary prevention refers to measures intended to avert the occurrence of disease. Secondary prevention refers to early diagnosis and prompt treatment in order to shorten the duration of illness, reduce symptoms, limit sequelae, and minimize contagion. Tertiary prevention refers to methods that limit disability and promote maximal physiological and psychological function in patients with diseases which cannot be reversed. Secondary and tertiary prevention are beyond the scope of this chapter.

PRIMARY PREVENTION

Measures for primary prevention fall into two categories: specific protection and health promotion. Specific protection is based on methods to prevent the occurrence of particular diseases by intercepting the specific cause of such diseases or by immunizing the population against the agents. The most spectacular example of success is the elimination of smallpox, a disease that 20 years ago afflicted as many as 15 to 20 million people, primarily in Third World countries, and had a 10–15 per cent mortality rate.[1] It is instructive to consider this example in greater detail because it is often taken as a prototype for preventive medicine.

What must be recognized is that smallpox is characterized by a set of unusual features: transmission is person-to-person and there is no known human carrier state—that is, a person who is asymptomatic but infectious; there is no known animal reservoir for the virus; patients are infectious only when the rash appears and only until the last scab has separated; immunity after vaccination or recovery from infection is long-lasting; furthermore, immune individuals can be recognized clinically by a life-long scar (post-vaccination or post-infection).

This unique combination of attributes made it possible to eliminate the disease from the face of the earth when three developments were put in place—(1) the production of a heat-stable freeze-dried vaccine which retained its potency in tropical countries, (2) a new public health strategy based on the isolation of identified cases and the prompt vaccination of all susceptible contacts, and (3) an international commitment to provide needed funding to the World Health Organization.

Immunization campaigns against other infectious diseases endemic in the population (such as diphtheria, pertussis, tetanus, rubella, rubeola and poliomyelitis) have also had substantial success in industrialized nations. But the goal of elimination continues to elude public health authorities because of lower immunogenicity of the vaccine, difficulty in detecting susceptibles by inexpensive methods, and the existence of latent periods when the patient is infectious but not clinically ill. These diseases continue to occur at high rates in the Third World because of problems in keeping the vaccine refrigerated, the lack of primary health care services for children, and the greater vulnerability of malnourished children to infectious diseases.

Immunization against communicable infectious diseases confers a benefit on the community as well as on the individual; susceptible persons who become ill serve as a source of infection for others. In most jurisdictions in the United States, proof of immunization is a condition for school entry; since schooling is compulsory, immunization against the common childhood diseases is in effect compulsory. This decision has been taken by duly elected governments in response to the unequivocal evidence of the extraordinary benefits for the community at large. However, all vaccines carry some risk for recipients. The question arises: what is the obligation of the state to the children (fortunately few in number) who suffer serious adverse outcomes? This matter is now a topic of public debate over proposals for federal insurance to cover the costs of care for such individuals. At present in the United States the only recourse for the family is to sue the manufacturer of the product. So costly have these suits become that some companies have abandoned the market, putting the supply of vaccines in some jeopardy.

The vaccine model has limited, if any, applicability to the non-infectious diseases which are now the major health problems in the industrialized world—heart disease, cancer, stroke, violence (accidents, homicide and suicide), and others. Multifactorial in causation, they are behaviourally mediated—that is, they occur at higher frequency in individuals who smoke, drink, overeat and engage in other health-injurious behaviours. With the possible exception of cancers of viral origin (and thus theoretically preventable by immunization), effective disease prevention demands major changes in life-style in the population, a considerably different challenge to public health measures than traditional immunization campaigns.

WHAT IS HEALTH PROMOTION?

Health promotion, in contrast to specific protection, refers to general measures which enhance host resistance to disease. Early in this century, Theobald Smith drew attention to host factors in disease:

> 'To learn that any given microbe which produced a well-defined disease in man is harmless to animals, that a disease germ, dangerous to one species, has no effect upon a closely related species, and that a human being may carry dangerous microbes which are held in check by unknown forces within him, are lessons which in themselves had a great influence in making medicine begin to appreciate the enormous complexity of the processes which protect us from disease or which lead to recovery.'[2]

Smith formulated a 'law of disease'—the likelihood of disease is directly proportional to the virulence of the provocative agent and inversely proportional to the resistance of the host.[3] This principle provides the scientific rationale for health promotion—namely, the enhancement of host factors that contribute to resistance to disease, whether or not the disease agents are known or controllable.

The provision of appropriate nutrition may be taken as the prototype of health promotion. Epidemiological studies of infection in infants and children demonstrate the following propositions: malnutrition increases the likelihood that exposure to infection will result in infectious disease; malnutrition impairs the individual's inflammatory and immune reactions to infectious disease; malnourished persons show increased systemic manifestation of diseases which tend to be more limited in those who are well nourished; in communities where malnutrition is prevalent, intercurrent infection and associated complications are markedly more frequent among the malnourished than the better nourished.[4]

In particular, gastrointestinal infection, made more likely by malnutrition, in itself increases the nutritional stresses on the host; fever adds to calorie requirements at the same time as infection decreases food intake and reduces the absorption of nutrients from the gut. Health may be further worsened by local customs of managing children with infectious diseases. In some pre-industrial societies, a diluted carbohydrate gruel (low in calories, proteins and electrolytes) is fed to sick children; the reduced food intake adds to the profound metabolic and electrolyte disturbances in the infected child.[4] Not only is immediate morbidity and mortality greater for malnourished infants and children, but longitudinal studies have demonstrated that the conjoining of chronic malnutrition with a disadvantaged home environment leads to retarded cognitive and social development.[5] Although nutrition is health promotion when the target is the reduction of the secondary complications associated with malnutrition, it is a specific preventive measure for malnutrition defined as a disease *per se*.

In contrast, the major problems of nutrition in the industrialized world are problems of overconsumption: too many calories (obesity) and too much fat (atherosclerosis). Is obesity a health problem? It is, according to a recent consensus conference convened by the United States National Institutes of Health.[6] Obesity is a risk factor for hypertension, diabetes, coronary artery heart disease and certain cancers; the greater the degree of overweight, the higher the excess death rate (in comparison to individuals in the normal weight range). Outcome studies indicate health benefits from weight reduction for patients with diabetes, hypertension, and hypercholesterolaemia. Reduction in the saturated fat content of the diet has been shown in some trials, but not in others, to improve the health status of individuals at risk for atherosclerotic heart disease.

THE COMPONENTS OF HEALTH PROMOTION

Measures to promote health can be divided into two broad categories: legislation and regulation to optimize the health-promoting features of the environment; health education and behaviour control to make health-promoting behaviours more likely and health injurious behaviours less likely.

The contrast between legislation and education may be exemplified by the methods to reduce injuries and fatalities from road traffic accidents. In the legislative category fall compulsory seat-belts laws, (thus far unsuccessful) efforts to make automatic air-bags mandatory in the production of cars, and highway safety engineering. In the second category are driver education courses for students. In between the two fall laws penalizing drunk driving and higher insurance premiums for drivers involved in accidents. In the first instance, the effort is to engineer an environment which will minimize the likelihood of bad outcomes even when the operator is at fault; in the second, the effort is to reduce human error by persuasion. In the intermediate instances, the expectation is that the threat of punishment will limit risk-taking behaviour.

Legislative measures remain controversial even when the evidence for effectiveness (as in the case of air-bags and seat-belts) is overwhelming. There is substantial opposition to controls on the lead content of petrol to reduce toxic emissions despite their success in lowering blood lead levels in children;[7] to fluoridation of the water supply to reduce the prevalence of dental caries; and to safety caps on bottles to minimize childhood poisonings. Despite the fact that these measures clearly improve the public health (and reduce expenditures for medical care), they are opposed on multiple grounds. These include costs (i.e., the increased price for the product or lowered profits for the producer); civil liberties (i.e., the 'right' to risk one's own health by not using belt or helmet); fears of toxicity (i.e., fluoride poisoning), and the like.

IS HEALTH PROMOTION A 'MODERN' INVENTION?

Campaigns to promote health by altering the behaviour of populations are often viewed as an unwarranted intrusion by the modern state into individual and family affairs. The assumption is that in earlier days and in 'simpler' societies, individuals and families were 'free' to make their own choices. To the contrary, the difference between past and present is a matter of having *more* information on which to make choices, choices which are, in any event, constrained by social forces as well as by the limitations on resources available to each family. Every human society, faced as all are by illness and death, elaborates theories of disease and of disease control.[8] These apply not only to methods of treatment but as well to measures to avoid becoming ill—including beliefs about proper diet, appropriate relations with other members of the community, taboos which must be observed, and magic rituals which must be followed. In preliterate societies, these 'health-promoting behaviours' are so thoroughly embedded in the culture of each society that they are not separable from everyday etiquette and religious ceremony.

Particularly ubiquitous are dietary prescriptions: for example, foods thought to be 'hot' or 'cold', with the balance between the two of great importance for the maintenance of health; substances to be avoided and others to be sought out to relieve certain symptoms of distress; foods with aphrodisiac properties and others more suitable for children or pregnant women or warriors. Some of these dietary regulations represent the distillation of folk wisdom—that is, the recognition of toxins, therapeutic substances, necessary dietary ingredients—and others have primarily a ritual function for group solidarity—that is, food avoidances imposed on adherent of religious groups such as Jews, Moslems and so on.

During the past two centuries, much of the improvement of health and the gain in longevity has come from increases in the standard of living of a population resulting from industrial development rather than by deliberate planned efforts on behalf of health. Mortality from tuberculosis fell by half between 1840 and 1880, two years before Koch discovered the tubercle bacillus. By 1940, it had fallen to one-sixth of that level, *well before doctors had an effective treatment*. Improved nutrition had increased host resistance; better housing and public health control measures had limited contagion.[9] Similar reductions in incidence of other infectious diseases have occurred well before the introduction of effective chemotherapy.[10] Another example of health benefits incidental to other purposes has been the introduction of 55 mile per hour speed limits on American motorways in response to the oil crisis; a measure undertaken on economic rather than public health grounds led to a measurable decrease in highway fatalities.

Yet this century has also seen an increase in mortality from coronary heart disease which has resulted from changes in life-style associated with modernization: a diet high in cholesterol and saturated fats (meat, eggs, and dairy products); an increasing proportion of cigarette smokers in the adult population; and a decline in levels of physical activity. Changing patterns of industrialization have been associated with the discharge of more pollutants into the environment—lead, asbestos, oxides of sulphur and nitrogen, among others—which have contributed to higher rates of cancer and chronic obstructive pulmonary disease. The point I emphasize is that all major changes in work patterns and life-styles have health consequences. This has always been true and will always be true. The present differs from the past only in two respects. The pace of change is much more rapid now and the systematic collection of public health information enables us to detect the effect of the changes and to design methods to reverse those which are undesirable.

Human life occurs only in a social context and that social context includes health beliefs. Those beliefs are inculcated into every child as that child learns the folkways of its own community. Health education is the contemporary version of this characteristic of earlier societies. It differs only to the extent that it is consciously identified and separated out of other educational measures, that it is based (to a greater or lesser extent) on systematic investigation of the effects of diet, exercise, and so on, that 'experts' are consulted in policy formulation, and that it is adopted after public debate by official bodies. This is not to imply that it is always effective or even sensible nor that it cannot be excessively intrusive. Nonetheless, it represents progress for public health to differentiate between tradition and ritual, on the one hand, and open evaluation of the health consequences of particular behaviours, on the other.

Decisions on public health programmes should be made only after full disclosure to the public of the benefits and disadvantages of the proposals and an opportunity for citizen input. Although sound programmes will be informed by careful weighing of the scientific evidence, the issues at stake in public policy almost always include value judgments as well as scientific judgments. Benefits and costs are rarely distributed symmetrically. When industrial plants discharge toxic effluents into the air, they pollute the air (a public good) for private gain.

Conversely, when health regulations impose emission controls on such plants, the citizenry at large benefits but the industry is at financial risk for the costs entailed and jobs for workers may be lost. All too often, the uncertainties in the scientific evidence (few matters are open and shut) are used by one side or the other to influence the decision under the guise of 'objective' scientific opinion.

PREVENTING CHILD ABUSE AND NEGLECT

When parents fail to provide adequate care for their children, how far is the state warranted in intervening to maintain the health of the child? If this principle applies in cases of physical abuse, is it proper in cases of emotional abuse and neglect?

In the United States, public law mandates the reporting of child abuse by health professionals. Moreover, it exempts them from civil action by aggrieved parents (unless malicious intent can be proved). Once the allegation has been reported to state welfare agencies, the complaint must be investigated and, if the evidence warrants, brought to the courts. The available legal options include mandatory counselling for parents if the situation is thought to be remediable; temporary removal of the child to a foster home if immediate danger threatens but there is hope of salvaging the home; and permanent foster care or adoption if the parents are held to be incorrigible. The Courts are charged with guaranteeing the rights of parents and children through due process.

Although child abuse and neglect can and do occur in all classes of society, they occur more frequently in families under severe social stress. Urban enclaves with a high frequency of child abuse are characterized by the aggregation of needy families competing for scarce resources in a 'neighbourhood' notably lacking in mutual support. Although clinical intervention can protect children when abuse has been diagnosed, care after the fact will at best have marginal effects on prevalence. Effective health promotion demands social action to mitigate the social conditions which make child abuse more likely.

If state action to intercept physical abuse is justified, does it apply to cases of emotional neglect and abuse? Every clinician has seen children whose emotional development has been stunted by the absence of affection, failure to respond to their needs, and rejecting and punitive parental attitudes. When parents request help, either for the child or for themselves, an ethical issue for the therapist arises only when treatment is terminated without resolution of the problem.

State intervention raises both legal and policy issues. From a legal standpoint, establishing a clear case for emotional neglect or abuse is often difficult. Whereas diagnostic physical stigmata result from violence, the psychiatric symptoms of the emotionally abused child do not in themselves establish criminal neglect as their cause. Courts are properly reluctant to rely on inferential evidence, in the absence of direct documentation of parental behaviour. Moreover, too low a threshold for intervention raises an important social policy question. The presumption in all societies is—and must be—that parents ordinarily act in the best interests of their children. That very expectation enhances parental responsibility. Too ready a resort to intrusion by the state weakens family ties and may make parents reluctant to seek help when a problem arises. Furthermore, alternative modes of care (foster care and group homes) are far from ideal. Disruption of the family unit is a risky step, one to be used only when the quality of the child's life in its own home seriously jeopardizes its development and is grossly inferior to available alternatives.

TO WHAT EXTENT IS THE ADOPTION OF HEALTH-PROMOTING BEHAVIOUR AN INDIVIDUAL RESPONSIBILITY OR A SOCIAL RESPONSIBILITY?

Because health damaging types of behaviour like smoking, overeating, drinking to excess and failure to exercise are exhibited by some people and not others, and because the diseases resulting from those behaviours put a sizeable burden for medical care costs on the entire community, measures to penalize such persons are being recommended with ever-greater frequency. Obviously, each individual does bear a responsibility for behaving prudently with respect to his or her own health; yet, the matter of equity must be raised before blaming the victim. There are marked differences in the prevalence of at risk behaviours by social class.

By the late 1960s, the United States death rate from coronary heart disease had risen to the second highest in the world; since that time, it has shown a steady and marked decline; currently the US rate is eighth among economically developed countries.[11] Over those 20 years, the proportion of cigarette smokers in the male population decreased steadily as did the *per capita* intake of food high in saturated fats; moreover, many more adults took up leisure-time exercise. With respect to all three life-styles, *the more educated changed more than the less educated*.

A recently reported data set from male employees of the DuPont Company revealed a greater rate of decline in the incidence of first acute myocardial infarctions and in case fatality rates among white collar employees than among production workers.[12] Among physicians, death rates from coronary heart disease fell from 15 per cent *higher* than that for age-matched men in the early 1950s to 31 per cent *lower* by the late 1970s. Trends in mortality from lung cancer among physicians parallel those for coronary heart disease. Whereas the majority of physicians, like men in the general population, were cigarette smokers in the 1950s, by the late 1970s rates for physicians were one-fourth those for the rest of the male population.[13]

Thus, although information about the health effects of smoking, diet and exercise have been available, at least in principle, to all Americans, the impact of that information has been far greater in changing behaviour among the more educated members of our population. Although the United States is a democratic society, opportunities for schooling and readiness to profit from that schooling are differentially distributed by the social class of the family.[14] Moreover, the availability of resources of time and money determine the ease or the difficulty with which the well-to-do and the poor are able to adopt healthy types of behaviour. Ubiquitous advertising campaigns by tobacco companies serve to confuse the less educated by casting doubt on the evidence connecting smoking with lung cancer. Thus, it is a gross injustice to hold the smoker solely responsible for his behaviour without taking into account the social pressures which make that behaviour more likely. Public health measures to contain or eliminate cigarette advertising, to end subsidies for tobacco farming, to increase taxes on cigarettes, and to capitalize on the success of school-based efforts at 'psychoimmunization' of youngsters against smoking are far more likely to reduce smoking rates than clinical measures directed at the individual. Indeed, Simon Chapman, of the Australian National Health and Medical Research Council, has argued for the abandonment of smoking cessation clinics because of a poor cost-benefit ratio, the greater efficiency of having general practitioners undertake such counselling, and the far greater importance of population-based methods.[15]

A particularly telling example of group effects on smoking behaviour is the fact that smoking rates have been increasing among young women in the United States at the very time that they have been decreasing among men. In consequence, deaths from lung cancer among women have exceeded deaths from breast cancer for the first time in our history![16] Many women have adopted a behaviour pattern once almost exclusively male, urged on by an insidious advertising campaign which implies—by means of the slogan 'You've come a long way, baby!' illustrated by graphics of women in new roles—that cigarette smoking is sophisticated modern behaviour by 'liberated' women.

Similar caveats about victim blaming apply to the current emphasis on programmes to reduce stress in the individual by relaxation methods (as opposed to attempts to alter the social conditions which give rise to stress). It is widely believed that stress is associated with coronary artery disease. The popular image is that the ambitious and over-worked executive is the prime target of coronary disease. Yet, data from the United Kingdom indicate a 26 per cent higher mortality from non-valvular heart disease in social class V relative to class I.[17] In a prospective study of 17 500 male London civil servants, the age-adjusted prevalence rates for cardiac mortality were 360 per cent higher among those in the lowest as contrasted with those in the highest employment grade.[18] These findings were confirmed in an American study of the prognosis for male survivors of acute myocardial infarction. The cumulative probability of death was *threefold higher* among those with less than a tenth grade education than it was among those with more than a high school education, after taking medical variables into account.[19] The investigators noted that 'the patients classified as being socially isolated and as having a high degree of life stress had more than four times the risk of death of the men with low levels of both stress and isolation.' Contrariwise, neither 'type A personality' nor depression proved to be a significant prognostic variable.[20] The incidence of coronary disease is almost twice as high among female clerical workers than among other women, with rates highest for those who had children and were married to blue collar workers.[21]

There are undoubtedly individual variations in susceptibility to stress-induced physiological strain. However, from the public health standpoint, the overriding imperative is to modify the social variables which overwhelm host resistance. The capacity of health care services to repair the wounded cannot keep pace with the rate at which casualties are generated by risk-taking behaviours. Syme[22] has calculated that it would take just about all available physician manpower in the United States to treat current coronary heart disease and to provide risk reduction programmes for those known to be at risk. Even if such measures were wholly successful (and unfortunately they are not), the campaign would be a failure because it would do nothing to limit the one million *new* persons entering the 'at risk' population each year.

None of this gainsays the value of health education but it argues for a broader conception of the content of that education than the contemporary emphasis on individual determinants of behaviour. And it implies that blaming the victim is a double injustice—it demeans those suffering from the consequences of health-injurious behaviours by adding feelings of guilt to their pain and it may rationalize denying care to them.

EVALUATION OF HEALTH PROMOTION

The evidence cited in this chapter that life-style is related to health status is generally accepted, though sceptics continue to point out that much of it is based on statistical association rather than unequivocal demonstrations of cause and effect by prospective studies. If there is no longer room for doubt about the causal role of smoking in lung cancer, coronary heart disease and chronic obstructive pulmonary disease, some uncertainty continues about the apparent association of atherosclerosis with diet and activity. There is, however, growing impatience with the insistence on meeting all the canons of scientific proof before taking public action, in view of staggering costs of medical care and the imperative to contain them. Whereas the use of randomized control trials is widely accepted as a necessary step in evaluating new medications, health promotion and education are often taken as having sufficient face validity to require no more than cursory evaluation, if any. This argument overlooks two hazards: one, that the measure may simply be ineffective (and thus represent an opportunity cost by wasting scarce resources) and that it may have unintended health hazards despite its plausibility.

During the 1960s, for example, when drug use was reaching epidemic proportions among adolescents and young adults in the United States, high school drug 'education' courses were introduced hastily in the hope of combating the epidemic. Unhappily, not only did such programmes fail to be effective, but in some studies they seemed to be associated with increased drug use.[23] A second set of issues has been raised by suggestive evidence that cholesterol lowering diets, recommended to control coronary heart disease, *may* be associated with increased rates of cancer.[24]

These few examples make evident the need for systematic evaluation of self-care protocols and health education measures before they are introduced on a wide scale.

BEHAVIOUR MODIFICATION

Methods of behavioural control are commonplace in every society, the clearest example being child-rearing practices which exert enormous pressure to bring the child into conformity with cultural norms. However, behaviour control in the modern sense refers to methods based on operant conditioning theory—the shaping of behaviour by controlling the contingencies of reinforcement. Its fundamental principle is that behaviour is maintained by its consequences. When a positive reinforcement (reward) follows a particular behaviour, the frequency with which that behaviour is manifested increases; when negative reinforcement (punishment) follows, its frequency decreases.

If a patient suffering from distressing symptoms seeks behaviour modification treatment, he or she contracts voluntarily to the reinforcement contingencies. So long as the choice is fully informed, there is no primary ethical problem about the treatment method itself, although the goals of treatment nonetheless merit examination. In contrast, serious ethical problems arise when behaviour modification methods are imposed on captive populations (prisoners, the institutionalized mentally ill or retarded, elderly patients in nursing homes, and the like). The 'treatment' is imposed on individuals who are not free to refuse. For many of them, informed consent cannot be obtained because of mental incompetence. Although prisoners may be intellectually capable of informed consent, by the nature of their imprisonment they are in no sense free to refuse because of institutional coercion. Under these conditions, a heavy burden of proof must be met that the institutional programme is indeed for the benefit of the subjects rather than the convenience of the caretakers.

To what extent can advertising be equated with behaviour modification? It is difficult to escape because it is omnipresent. It operates for the benefit of the sellers rather than the consumers and owes no allegiance to truth in any reasonable definition of that term. It is designed to modify the behaviour of consumers, not only by propaganda in favour of the product, but also by associating the use of the product with attributes (beauty, masculinity, wealth, and so on) entirely irrelevant to the product but attractive to the buyer. It differs significantly from the operant model in that the link between the behaviour (buying) and the reinforcer (advertising) is reversed.

Consumer advocates point out that advertising is used deliberately to induce the purchase of products which injure health—cigarettes, alcohol, 'empty calorie' foods and so on. Public health arguments for banning such advertising are countered by concerns over the restriction of free speech. It is contended that, however well-intentioned, limitation on what can be presented to the public will lead inevitably to the loss of a right no less valuable than health. Yet, as Justice Holmes of the United States Supreme Court pointed out many years ago, the right to free speech does not include the right to yell out 'fire!' in the middle of a crowded auditorium because of the clear and present danger to life it would entail. There is a delicate balance which must be weighed between the right to health and the right to speech.

The alternative to banning the advertising of products injurious to health is the provision of time for countervailing educational 'advertising'. This proposition faces a serious practical problem: the disproportion between the budgets controlled by commercial interests and those available to consumer groups. Balance might be obtained if government tax funds (from taxes on the product, for example) were to be used for health education.

RECONCILING THE IRRECONCILABLE: FAMILY PLANNING POLICY AND THE RIGHT TO HAVE CHILDREN

No single issue which affects the health of the population highlights the tension between the personal rights and the civic duties of citizens more sharply than the demographic imperative which drives family planning policy in the People's Republic of China. Traditional Chinese culture valued fecundity in marriage highly with particular emphasis on the bearing of many sons. The Confucian ethic of venerating parents and elders was reflected in a classic definition of bliss: 'five generations living together'. The cultural imperative for large families can be regarded as functional during millenia when infant mortality rates were high; the likelihood of having children survive into adulthood as a source of care for elderly parents was the greater the larger the family. The problem for modern China is precisely the opposite. Success in reducing infant mortality has created enormous population pressures on limited resources; controlling population size has become a major concern of social policy. This brings the state into conflict with the wishes of parents who, reflecting traditional values, continue to want to have large families. If decisions are left to individual sets of parents, the welfare of the nation is put in jeopardy. If a draconian state policy enforces rigid limitations on family size, the rights of families are abrogated.

It is instructive to compare current population data for the People's Republic of China and the United States. The 1982 Chinese census tabulated a total of just over 1 008 000 000 people on mainland China, some 22 per cent of the world's population! In mid-1982, the population of the United States was estimated by the Bureau of the Census at about 232 million.[25] The land mass of China is approximately the same as that of the United States (including Alaska and Hawaii), but only about 10 per cent of the Chinese land mass is suitable for cultivation whereas the corresponding figure for the United States is 21 per cent. Thus, the amount of arable land per head in China is less than one-ninth that in the United States—and less than one-third of the world average. The magnitude of the social problem constituted by population growth in China is epitomized in the following straightforward projection: by the year 2000, the Chinese population will have *grown by 200 million persons, even if* present family planning policy is moderately successful. The People's Republic of China will have to provide food, clothing, housing, education, health care, transportation and other social necessities for a *new* population about equivalent to that of the United States.

In part, the dilemma facing China results from its remarkable accomplishments. As a result of a general improvement in living standards and effective public health measures, the crude death rate[26] has fallen from 25.8 per thousand in 1953 to 7.9 in 1982. In parallel, life expectancy at birth has risen from 40 to almost 65 years. The birth rate in China declined by half between 1954 and 1961, jumped tremendously between that year and 1963 (from 19 to 44 per thousand) and then began a slow decline: to 34 by 1970, to 23 by 1975 and to 17 in 1980. As the result of a high birth rate in the face of a declining death rate, the rate of natural increase peaked at 34 per 1000 in 1963 and then declined slowly to 11 per 1000 in 1980.

Changes in birth rate have geometric rather than arithmetic consequences. The word 'momentum' is employed in demography to refer to the tendency of a population to keep increasing long after its high birth rates have fallen. Population increase will continue for about 50 years after the decline of birth rate to replacement levels. Data from the People's Republic of China indicate that the number of births peaked at 29 million in 1963 and were as high as 27 million in 1970. The 1982 census revealed that there had been almost 21 million births in 1981.[27] The large number of births in the 1960s and the early 1970s have resulted in large cohorts of women who will be in their maximum period of fertility in the 1980s and 1990s.

The 'one child family' slogan was introduced in 1979 in recognition of the consequences of the large number of births in the 1960s and 1970s. The decision was taken despite awareness of its demographic consequences: the aging of the population; foreseeable shortages of labour and of men of military age in the next generation; unbalanced sex ratios; and the problem that each young couple would have to support four parents and one child. Speaking for the government of the People's Republic of China, Yu Zhenpeng and Chen Siyi wrote:

> 'Calling on each couple to have one child is the best choice we can make in solving the present population problem of our country. This alternative has its drawbacks, but the drawbacks are only temporary. Moreover, since we are aware of them, we can take prompt action to solve many of the difficulties. The drawbacks are insignificant compared with the problems that would arise if the four modernizations were delayed by excessive growth in population.'[28]

Access to effective methods of contraception and of sterilization are universal in China (or as nearly so as they can be made in so vast a nation), with abortion in extensive use for back-up in the event of failed or omitted contraception. Not only is there extensive official propaganda in favour of family limitation but the fertility status of women is monitored on a mandatory basis by neighbourhood units in many communes. If a second pregnancy is discovered, abortion is 'strongly encouraged' by official policy. In communes zealous about meeting birth quotas, 'strongly encouraged' in effect means compulsory. Official exemptions to one-child policy are made in instances where the first child is mentally or physically disabled, where the father is an only child, for members of minority populations, and for fishermen or farmers in less fertile mountain areas where the first child is a daughter.

Official data from Chinese sources[27] reveal a large variation between one city and another and between urban and rural areas in the percentage of married couples who say they would be willing to have only one child. The New York Times (10/9/83) quoted Qian Xinzhong, the Minister in charge of the State Family Planning Commission, as stating:

> 'There are certain districts where family planning programmes are very well accepted. But also there are districts where family planning is not very successful. The good places are really good and the bad places are really bad.'

An important element in the difference between urban and rural attitudes (80 per cent of the population is rural) towards rearing children is the fact that it costs a family almost four times as much to rear a child in urban areas; furthermore, children begin to contribute to family income at a much earlier age in farm districts. This urban/rural differential in attitudes has been compounded by the introduction of the 'responsibility system', a policy which permits farm families to retain the profits from production exceeding the quotas set as norms. This has, on the one hand, led to a very substantial improvement in the productivity of Chinese agriculture. On the other, it increases the incentive for the couple to have more children; a larger family can produce more crops and earn greater profits.

The measures the People's Republic of China has introduced sharply reduce freedom of choice for the individual, a value held high in the West but one which throughout the millenia of Chinese history has been available only to the privileged few. Given the economic consequences of the population explosion which resulted from the failure of social policy during the 1960s and 1970s, social necessity demands an effective family planning policy if China is to avoid famine and impoverishment. In the words of Qian Xinzhong: 'Giving birth to children is not just a family affair. It also has an effect on the future of nations'.

In the United States and Japan, smaller families and larger numbers of elderly place traditional patterns of care for dependent elderly persons in jeopardy. Whereas in the past the extended family took care of its own elderly, more of them, especially those aged over 75 years, are being moved into old age homes and into nursing homes supported by public funds. The fact that this change is taking place in Japan, where tradition demands a filial devotion to the care of parents and grandparents akin to that of Chinese culture, predicts a like secular phenomenon in China. In China, the anxieties of the elderly have been increased since the Cultural Revolution which led to a decline in respect for the elderly. One official report on rural reactions to the one child policy acknowledged that: 'They worry about who will take care of them in their old age'.[29] Peasants express alarm that 'many young people are unfilial' and that 'the old, the weak, and the women often get the worst of the deal'.[30]

Reduced family size has marked effects on the life cycle of women. At the turn of this century, in the United States, life expectancy for women was just under 50 years. If a woman continued to have children into her 30s, as the majority did, almost all of her adult life was occupied by her maternal role. Currently, female life expectancy in the United States is just under 80 years and fertility rates are just about half of what they were at the turn of the century. Today, more than half of a woman's adult lifetime takes place *after* her children have become adults themselves. Moreover, in the United States, among married women aged 30–34 years, the percentage who had only one birth has increased from 12 to 18 per cent in the last decade[31] and current data indicate that as many as 20 to 25 per cent of women will remain childless.[32] Equality for women in all spheres of society has always been a fundamental human right; today, it is a matter of social necessity as well. Each society needs the full contribution of all its citizens.

In almost all societies, it has been traditional to prefer the birth of a son to the birth of a daughter. However, in an industrial society, the preference for male children is anachronistic. In rural communities, cultural preference for sons accords with a realistic economic analysis of family consequences. So marked are the differences between the ways boys and girls are cared for that the sex differences in child mortality in the West (higher among males) are reversed in many developing countries.[33] Lincoln Chen and his colleagues have undertaken a series of studies in Bangladesh in an effort to analyse the reasons for the high female mortality.[34] When nutritionists measured the food served at family meals, they found that mothers gave more of what little food there was to their sons than to their daughters. Families also differed in the way they used health care for sons and daughters. Since health care is difficult to obtain, because of the distance to be travelled to reach a clinic, the decision to bring a child in for care represents expenditure of scarce resources. Sick male children are more often brought to the clinic than sick female children.

In its official pronouncements, the government of the People's Republic of China labels female infanticide as an intolerable crime; its newspapers publicize severe punishment for those found guilty. For example, the People's Daily, on 7 April 1983 reported the drowning of 40 baby girls in 1980 and 1981 by members of a single production team in Anhui Province. The same newspaper, a month earlier, had quoted a spokesperson of the Federation of Women's Associations as stating: 'Drowning and killing of girl infants and the maltreatment of mothers of infant girls have become a grave social problem'. The disproportionate ratio of males to females in the child population of some rural areas indicates either substantial rates of female infanticide or the under-reporting of live female children (in order to escape the economic penalties for having a second child).

ETHICS IN CONTEXT

The Chinese example makes evident the major consequences of family planning policy for all sectors of society. Not only are the rights of parents directly affected in the first instance, but a wave of secondary effects spreads throughout the community—on the status of the elderly, on sex ratios in the population, on the role of women, on the burden on the working population for the support of dependents, and so on, leaving no major component of the society unaffected. Given the population explosion of the post-war period in China and the limitations on natural resources, it is difficult to see how any government, of whatever political persuasion could fail to intervene forcefully with the survival of the population taking precedence over individual rights. Similar decisions are likely to force themselves on other governments in the Third World; India's population, now 750 million, may well exceed that of China early in the next century if present rates of increase continue, with explosive political consequences. Western European nations, on the other hand, now face birth rates lower than replacement levels—that is, the populations have begun to decline in number as well as to increase in age. Not surprisingly, pro-natalist movements have grown in strength, partly on grounds of national chauvinism. This is evident in France where fears of being once again overwhelmed by Germany have been explicitly acknowledged as arguments in favour of policies to increase the birth rate.

Ethical judgments in the two sectors of the world rest on fundamentally different premises. The industrialized nations can allow themselves to emphasize the rights of individuals to make decisions about procreation; they face no immediate crises and consequently can employ education and tax policy for longer term readjustments. Relying on such strategies with their inherent time lag and low efficiency is to invite disaster in countries hardly able to feed their populations and often not at all able to do so without major infusions of foreign aid (with its inevitable limitations on national sovereignty).

Western societies emphasize personal autonomy as a central ethical principle. That stance has arisen in the context of high levels of economic development and the evolution of stable political democracies over the centuries. It is the height of arrogance to use our standards to pass judgment on societies which stand in relationship to our present economic good fortune as did the West many centuries ago. What we can—and should—do is to assist Third World countries to move rapidly through the cycle of development which we have undergone in order that they, too, can attain the affluence necessary for the enjoyment of the rights we prize so highly.

REFERENCES

1. Breman, J. C. and Arita, I. Confirmation and maintenance of smallpox eradication. *N Engl J Med* 1980; **303**: 1263–73.
2. Smith, T. Quoted in Beecher, H. K. and Altschule, M. D. *Medicine at Harvard: the first 300 years*. Hanover, New Hampshire: University Press of New England, 1977.
3. Gage, S. H. Theobald Smith 1859–1934. *Cornell Vet* 1935; **25**: 207–228.
4. Birch, H. G. and Cravioto, J. Infection, nutrition and environment in mental development. **In**: *The Prevention of Mental Retardation through Control of Infectious Diseases*. Washington, DC, PHS Publication No 1692, 1966: pp. 227–248.
5. Richardson, S. A. The relation of severe malnutrition in infancy to the intelligence of school children with different life histories. *Pediatric Res* 1976; **10**: 57–61.
6. National Institutes of Health Consensus Development Conference Statement. *Health Implications of Obesity*. Mimeographed, Washington, National Institutes of Health, 11–13 February 1985.
7. Centers for Disease Control. Blood-lead levels in US population. *Morb Mort Weekly Rep* 1982; **31**: 132–134.
8. Eisenberg, L. The physician as interpreter: ascribing meaning to the illness experience. *Comp Psychiat* 1981; **22**: 239–248.
9. McKeown, T. M. *The Role of Medicine: Dream, Mirage or Nemesis*. London: Nuffield Provincial Hospitals Trust, 1976.
10. Kass, E. H. Infectious diseases and social change. *J Infect Dis* 1971; **123**: 1010–1014.
11. Stamler, J. The marked decline in coronary heart disease mortality rates in the United States, 1968–1981: summary of findings and possible explanations. *Cardiology* 1985; **72**: 11–22.
12. Pell, S. and Fayerweather, W. E. Trends in the incidence of myocardial infarction and in associated mortality and morbidity in a large employed population, 1957–1983. *New Engl J Med* 1985; **312**: 1005–1011.
13. Enstrom, J. E. Trends in mortality among California physicians after giving up smoking 1950–1979. *Brit Med J* 1983; **286**: 1101–1105.
14. Eisenberg, L. and Earls F. J. Poverty, social depreciation and child development. **In**: Hamburg D.A. (ed). *American Handbook of Psychiatry*. Vol VI. New York: Basic Books, 1975: 275–291.
15. Chapman, S. Stop-smoking clinics: a case for their abandonment. *Lancet 1985*; **1**: 918–920.

16. Correa, P. and Zavala, D. E. Letter to the editor. Lung Cancer: leading cause of cancer deaths in Louisiana white females. *J Natl Cancer Institute* 1984; **72**: 1–2.
17. Rose, G. and Marmot, M. G. Social class and coronary disease. *Br Heart J* 1981; **45**: 13–19.
18. Marmot, M. G., Shipley, M. J. and Rose, G. Inequalities in death specific explanations of general patterns. *Lancet* 1984; **1**: 1003–1006.
19. Weinblatt, E., Ruberman, W., Goldberg, J. *et al*. Relation of education to death after myocardial infarction. *New Engl J Med* 1978; **299**: 60–65.
20. Ruberman, W., Weinblatt, E., Goldberg, J. D. and Chaudhary, B. Psychosocial influences on mortality after myocardial infarction. *New Engl J Med* 1984; **311**: 552–559.
21. Haynes, S. G., Feinlieb, M. Women, work and coronary heart disease. *Am J Pub Hlth* 1980; **70**: 133–141.
22. Syme, S. L. Social support and risk reduction. *Moebius* 1984; **4**: 44–53.
23. Durell, J. and Bukoski, W. Preventing substance abuse: the state of the art. *Public Health Rep* 1984; **99**: 23–31.
24. Ederer, F., Leren, P., Turpeinen, O. and Frantz, I. Cancer among men on cholesterol lowering diets: experiences from five clinical trials. *Lancet* 1971; **2**: 203–206.
25. Bureau of the Census. Population profile of the United States: 1982. Current Population Reports; Special Studies, Series P-23, No. 130, December 1983.
26. Banister, J. An analysis of recent data on the population of China. *Population and Development Review* 1984; **10**: 241–271.
27. Tien, H. Y. China: demographic billionaire. Population Reference Bureau April/1983; **38**, No. 2.
28. New China News Agency. 2 October 1980.
29. People's Daily, Beijing. 2 September 1980.
30. Sha Anxi Noagmin Bao. 7 January 1981.
31. US Bureau of the Census. Current Population Reports, Series P-20, Number 341, Table 7, p. 34, 1979 (October).
32. Bloom, D. E. What's happening to the age at first birth in the United States? A study of recent cohorts. *Demography* 1982; **19**: 351–370.
33. D'Souza, S. and Chen, L. C. Sex differentials in mortality in rural Bangladesh. *Population and Development Review* 1980; **6**: 257–270.
34. Chen, L. C., Huq, E. and D'Souza, S. Sex bias in the family allocation of food and health care in rural Bangladesh. *Population and Development Review* 1981; **7**: 55–70.

Ethical Dilemmas in Health Promotion
Edited by S. Doxiadis

CHAPTER 10

Health Economics and Ethics

MARTINE BUNGENER

SUMMARY

This chapter looks at the place of health economics in prevention and examines five difficulties in evaluating the economic effectiveness of preventive strategies. It also underlines the economic paradox of prevention which appears to result inevitably—at least for a preliminary period—in an increase in people's consumption of curative medicine and thus in an increase in expenditure on health. In the current economic climate, the economist must play a part in planning prevention and health care where difficult ethical choices have to be made but economic criteria must never stand alone. The basic choices must be political and democratic but both economics and medicine provide the means for implementing these decisions.

INTRODUCTION

The ethical aspects of the economics of prevention combine questions of economics proper and the issues discussed in depth throughout this book on medical ethics and prevention.

The first issue is the relevance of the tool of economics to the medical debate. The cost of medical care has increased greatly over the last few decades. In many countries, all or part of this cost is financed by the community and this requires attention to the best possible allocation of the resources available. This question comes within the scope of the economist whose skills can help to advise on the best distribution of available wealth. However, economists are not expected to define the objectives of prevention, and it is here that the economist's perspective must admit its ethical limitations. Once the objective has been defined, the economist's task is to suggest the most financially valid solutions, to allow the objectives set to be attained at the lower possible cost. It is obvious, however, that there is a flaw in this analysis since, given the current state of western economies, we cannot define objectives without reference to some sort of economic rationale. Financial criteria must intervene in the actual definition of the objectives, and even in the decision to choose one objective in preference to another. The crucial ethical question remains whether it is legitimate to use economic criteria to define certain objectives, and the relative importance which such criteria have or should have in terms of political decision-making.

In the context of prevention, objectives must be orientated towards health. But they cannot be easily defined since the goal is to achieve the most satisfactory state of health possible within the reality of limited financial resources. This is the proper objective of health economics. In curative medicine, the economist's role is a secondary one since therapeutic action is largely dictated by the techniques and pharmaceutical products available to the medical profession. Even here, however, we must not underestimate the contribution a quantitative approach has made to medical efficiency. The economist, having provided the doctor with an economic dimension—notably perhaps in cost-benefit analysis—has helped him to improve treatment.

A difference arises in considering preventive rather than curative action since this implies defining a strategy from among several possibilities, the most extreme being to do nothing at all. It is obvious that here the economist has an essential role and that economic thinking about prevention has undergone various modifications because of the particular difficulties encountered in the debate.

In this chapter, I propose to look at the continuing debate and the difficulties it raises with the aim of emphasizing the economic paradox and the question of ethical limitations. This approach also emphasizes the need to rescue health economics from becoming engulfed in moral discussions since the very survival of medical effectiveness is at stake in a context of diminishing resources.[1]

The ethical limitations of the economics of prevention may well be found at the level of the decision-making processes for defining public health policy, and the place which it should occupy within these processes. Nevertheless we cannot deny the validity of the economic tool in the prevention debate.[2]

THE CONTINUING DEBATE ON PREVENTION

Promoting preventive action implies the availability of information on the anticipated results; the information is obviously mainly medical in nature, but the expected benefits to health must also be examined in relation to the means by which they are achieved. In the last instance, the common denominator of this comparison, and perhaps the earliest to grasp, is the financial factor.

Thus, discussions bearing on the health effectiveness of prevention cannot be treated in isolation from discussions concerning its economic effectiveness, even where this relationship is contradicted by an *a priori* statement that the aim of prevention is not to reduce health expenditure, and that no proof has even been provided of such an effect. The relationship can more truthfully be described as one of interdependence. The question of the economic effectiveness of prevention depends largely on information about its medical effects. Where these cannot be easily demonstrated, economic criteria take on added importance.

Two examples of problems which are amenable to prevention—the health effects of cigarette smoking and perinatal abnormalities—demonstrate the issues involved. The evidence for improvements in health and reduction in morbidity and mortality which result from stopping smoking is clear. Furthermore an economic analysis for Northern Ireland (population 1.5 million), including all measurable factors, showed that while the economic gains from cigarette consumption measured £117.3 million, the actual cost to the population in mortality and morbidity substantially exceeded this sum, giving a net cost to the Northern Ireland economy of £103 million.

In the other example, although the effects of better monitoring during pregnancy should clearly lead to the reduction in birth abnormalities and premature births, the direct causal and economic relationships are difficult to determine with any real exactitude. Apart from the immediate cost of complicated labour and delivery and the specific medical care required by premature babies, how do we evaluate the advantage, in economic terms, for the mother, the child, and society?

In general, the full economic impact of sickness and health remains a matter of delicate and complicated appraisal. At first sight it might appear relatively easy to draw up and cost a table of material resources allocated to the health system for prevention of sickness, and improvement or restoration of health.[3] These resources may be identified and accounted for in terms of personnel employed or the purpose for which they are employed, even if in terms of marginal accounting it is less easy to determine the extent to which these resources are spent on curing illness. However, many more elusive elements—potential wasted through illness or gained because of its non-appearance or disappearance, in terms of productivity or social and family activities—also enter into play, and although they are difficult to evaluate they cannot be ignored. Identification of the potential gained through successful preventive actions implies a belief in a world in which sickness will either disappear or at least diminish, and history has shown this to be a myth. How can we then evaluate in economic terms and make the best use of the potential which would result from a state of improved public health, and integrate its effects into population statistics and statistics on national productivity? In other words, how do we evaluate the cost of human life?[4]

The very wording of this question suggests the extraordinary ambition of such enquiries given the weakness of their theoretical and ethical bases. Nonetheless there are reports of economic surveys which attempt to cost losses in productivity, domestic activity or leisure as a result of sickness as a way of justifying the allocation of expenditure on prevention. Fortunately this practice has not been extended to curative medicine.

Thus we can see the inadequacy of the economic concept of 'cost' when applied to sickness, and how it can lead to debatable analyses, if the economist does not refer to ethical and moral principles as a way of limiting his intervention. The neutral notion of costs, in terms of resources allocated, can be extended improperly to arrive at a standardized notion of burdens which weigh too heavily on the community and which total or partial disappearance of the illness concerned would reduce. In the case of prevention the danger is quite obvious.

This notion appears even more improper when we consider that it is difficult to ignore phenomena of economic shift or shifts in the sickness ratio. Whether we are discussing marginal economics or a more straightforward hypothesis of reduction, we do not know the laws governing evolution of costs related to sickness. Under these conditions, hypotheses of proportionality are quite obviously extremely imprecise, and may even falsify the decision-making process on which they are intended to throw light. The notion of costs and calculation of costs are not so much debatable in themselves as in the distortions and misinterpretations to which they may lead. However this must not force the decision-maker to come to the conclusion that calculating the costs of the measures put into practice is a useless activity.[5]

If we make allowance for these factors, qualitative and quantitative knowledge of the phenomena generated by preventive measures may well help in reaching more rational decisions. However before such empirical knowledge and the associated calculations can be put to use, a number of difficulties must be overcome.

DIFFICULTIES IN EVALUATING THE ECONOMIC EFFECTIVENESS OF PREVENTION

From the outset, the difficulties are intensified by the diversity of the terms used to describe the notion of 'effectiveness'. In French we use two terms: effectiveness (*efficacité*) and advantage (*avantage*) which implies a less positive judgment.[6]

Advantage covers any normally favourable effect felt by an individual or a group, usually linked to the use of goods and services at their disposal. In this sense, it may be quantified. Effectiveness, on the other hand, covers a much wider field in that certain results may be quite obviously attained but are very difficult to translate into figures.

The difference between the two terms forms the basis for two different methods: 'cost-effectiveness' methods which measure the results obtained against the means employed without necessarily quantifying them, and 'cost-advantage' methods which attempt to quantify the expected results according to a variety of qualitative, quantitative and financial criteria.

In English there are three specific terms for use in this debate—'efficacy', 'effectiveness' and 'efficiency'— which allows a more subtle appraisal of a situation generally agreed to be a very complex one. To 'efficacy'—the capability of producing the desired effect—we add the notion of 'effectiveness', which implies a definite modification of the natural course of a disease or illness, and 'efficiency' which remains qualitative in meaning. 'Efficiency' does have a literal translation in French (*efficience*), but it is a term which is rarely used in the prevention debate. However, beyond these subtleties of language, we must still deal with the question of how to measure the results obtained or anticipated. Here we encounter five orders of difficulty.

First Difficulty: Choosing the Reference Situation

Effectiveness implies that a change has been brought about in the course of events and that it can be positively evaluated. And evaluating a change implies the existence of a generally accepted reference situation. However we are faced with a dilemma in the case of prevention. Should this reference situation be chosen on medical, economic or even socio-political grounds?

The economic reference, as any cost argument, cannot be used in isolation. Even where it may appear watertight, the fact that calculations suggest a certain profitability does not mean that implementation of the particular action will necessarily give the expected results. The same type of argument can be used where the reference is essentially medical, since here too the result may be compromised by resistance from individuals or institutions, and the length of time it takes for new structures or new practices to be disseminated. Thus social or political factors, and the potential receptivity of the population to the measures advocated will play an important part in determining final results. In fact actual results may differ markedly from those anticipated to the extent that in some cases the opposite effect is created. Promoters of health education campaigns are less afraid that their action will be ineffective than that it will be misunderstood.

To avoid creating the opposite effect from that originally intended, we must state clearly the goal of the preventive action to be undertaken. Are we aiming to make financial savings in the case of obvious abuse, or to improve the state of the public health and reduce the frequency of certain diseases, or do we intend a combination of these two expectations? And by improving the state of health of a group or a population, are we attempting to improve individual wellbeing or obtain increased productivity for society? Unless we make a clear statement of the goal to be pursued, which implies a predetermined reference situation, it is impossible to evaluate any improvements made or advantages gained. Even then we must take care that this advantage or benefit does not generate negative effects, which remain wholly or partially without compensation in related systems—in other words, that they do not have iatrogenic effects either medically or socially. The line separating the medical and social spheres is thin and porous, and any medical or preventive action must be considered in the context of society.

Second Difficulty: Estimating Needs

This problem is to some extent related to the first since a given need exists within a system of social and medical references without which it would not exist and which gives it meaning. When defining a need for preventive actions we meet the same difficulties as for any other health need, since such actions must be seen in the light of a whole system of attitudes, perceptions and behavioural patterns which cannot be understood solely in medical terms. However, if we compare the health situation of different social groups, we can sidestep the difficulty of immediate evaluation of needs as such, since this will reveal the more flagrant inequalities which it would seem moral to attempt to reduce. Equally we cannot ignore the difficulty of distinguishing between medical and social needs which is intensified in the field of prevention because of our realization that social and life-style factors are also risk factors.

Third Difficulty: What Are We Evaluating and How?

These central questions are crucial here. Having recognized these risks of potential error, the economist's task is still to produce figures. In the field of health, his job is to decide what should be measured and the scale of values to be used. When we are dealing with actions or tangible facts, we may use a readily available scale such as the cost of a particular treatment or the remuneration of qualified personnel. Subsequently we need only make allowances for technical factors such as inflation, for relative prices, quantifying in terms of volume or value, for deductions for depreciation, and separation of capital costs and operating costs. When we try to measure behavioural patterns or human feelings, such as suffering prevented, improved quality of life and so on, the procedures are extremely delicate. Nevertheless it is quite legitimate to take these factors into account. Even when we try to express them quantitatively—that is, number of days saved or gained—can we usefully compare the days of a child with those of an adult or an old person, to mention biological differences only, and without going into cultural or socio-economic differences?

Do we not after all find ourselves suggesting, albeit indirectly, some sort of statistical approximation of the value of human life? In spite of the possibility of confusing the cost of the illness with the cost of the efforts to deal with it and of all the difficulties and complexities of calculation, we come back frequently to this concept of the 'cost of a human life' in terms of our efforts to protect it, prolong it, or even begin it. In some cases, this figure may be deduced from political decisions. The launch of a programme to improve roads or crossroads, for example, with the justification of the number of accidents which will therefore be avoided, allows us to attribute a financial value to each accident avoided. This value can then be used as a reference for other investments or to reveal disparities inherent in prevention policies carried out in other sectors, and the different figures given by other investments in the field of industrial safety or repair of damage caused by accidents.

These methods of calculation lead us in effect to figures whose limits lie anywhere between 50 000 and 335 000 French francs when it is a question of routine screening and between 3000 and 85 000 French francs for the prevention of childhood illnesses.[7] An average figure of 150 000 French francs was proposed in France in 1972 but was never used.[8] A study in 1977[9] and the report of a British conference in 1982[10] emphasized the wide variety of results in any attempts to quantify the value of human life. Quite apart from the method of calculation, the diversity of the various elements involved explains the width of the boundaries that we can attempt to set. It is also the case that the cost of care and other specific interventions will represent between a fifth and a tenth of the estimated figures. We are now dealing with an ethical question. How can we justify the discrepancies observed in such calculations and how can we test their validity?

On a more technical level, when making evaluations of this type, the economist must avoid drawing hasty conclusions, or over-simplifying the problem by comparing factors which are not comparable, such as the cost of medical care and the reduction of pain. No economic principle can be put forward to justify such practices.

Fourth Difficulty: Individual Versus Community Effectiveness

The different characteristics of the diseases or risks which we wish to prevent imply a choice between factors of risk for the individual or the community as a whole. In other words, we seek either to encourage a particular type of individual behaviour, or to lay down measures for the good of the community. Thus, according to the type of prevention agreed upon, the cost may be expressed in the form of individual investment, as in the case of the campaign to combat cigarette smoking, or group consumption. Preventive campaigns aimed at the community may be further categorized according to whether the results can be broken down and expressed in terms of individual investment, such as compulsory vaccination, or not, as in the case of fluoridation of the water supply.[11] The desired effects may also be classified in terms of personal results and community protection. But they are not necessarily cumulative and may even prove to be contradictory.

It is obvious that prevention which is effective on the individual level is not necessarily effective for the community as a whole, because of the unjustifiable increase in expenditure which it would represent. As proof of this fact we might cite routine general health check-ups, a programme which is not economically unfeasible. We also meet a moral problem in this area which we cannot hope to solve from economic data alone—that is, the prevention of rare diseases. This type of action would commit large sums of money to campaigns which would benefit a very small number of people.

The inverse situation also creates a difficult ethical problem. Effective community prevention occasionally has serious iatrogenic effects on certain individuals.[12] Here we are faced with a moral problem just as serious as the first, which balances the protection of a majority of individuals against the risks for a small minority. In this case the interests of the community are in direct opposition to those of a few individuals. A well-known example of this state of affairs was the use of 'primaquine' to combat malaria in California which caused some members of the black community to develop serious anaemia. A biological solution was eventually found which made it possible to identify the subjects at risk and to exclude them from the community prevention campaign.[13]

These examples are obviously extreme, but they do illustrate a situation which arises frequently in the field of economics— the 'gap' between micro-economic results and macro-economic effects. There is no immediate relationship between micro-economic methods and macro-economic results. Different factors are at work in each situation, and in economic terms we find the same kind of incompatibility which sometimes exists between simple individual preventive measures and group rejection or failure to understand such measures. We must also take into account factors concerning social and economic permissiveness, and receptivity to or diversion, even the complete transformation of individual measures when adapted to the scale of the community. For neither economic structures nor human groups are passive, and they may give rise to unforeseen diversions or transfers when the scale is modified. What may be tolerable for some individuals may cease to be tolerable for the community as a whole. We cannot therefore rely on a process of calculation based on simple combinations of different data.

The 'micro-macro' debate is aggravated by the fact that economic feasibility must be evaluated within a framework of inelastic global expenditures allocated to health service activity as a whole for both preventive and curative medicine, which is then distributed between the different programme by means of a series of micro-economic decisions.

Making decisions implies a distribution of resources which itself implies choosing certain actions to the detriment of others. This makes the question of effectiveness even more problematical. Wrong choices result not only in a relative non-effectiveness, but also cancel out another choice which would have had effective results of some sort or another, and these have to be taken into account. However the question of the best choice brings up yet another dilemma.

Fifth Difficulty: The Long-Term/Short-Term Dilemma

The economic effectiveness of prevention is presented diagrammatically as an immediate expense which will obviate the need for later expenditure on curative medical care. The seeming simplicity of this equation conceals a more complex reality, both from the economic and the medical point of view.

The economic question is a well-known theoretical problem to which are attached a number of empirical solutions, since it is inherent in any investment choice. The economic validity of such choices is identified by using a suitable rate of actualization. This rate makes it possible to compare the economic and financial 'yield' of different investments over different time periods corresponding to very different categories of life expectancy. Using this rate in preventive decisions allows us to compare the saving of a human life tomorrow with that which will be saved a generation later, and thus justifies the cost of basic research compared to applied research or immediate experimentation.

There is, however, also another problem encountered by those responsible for investment decisions concerned with preventive health measures—this is the strict financial feasibility of health expenditures. Such investment may have the effect of keeping alive individuals who will later fall sick again and will in the future consume medical care which would not have been necessary had the individual died earlier. However, although this statement may make sense in economic terms, it is ethical nonsense and demonstrates the limitations of using economic arguments in the debate on preventive processes. Nevertheless it does hint at a paradoxical economic aspect of prevention which has some validity.

THE ECONOMIC PARADOX OF PREVENTION

Prevention covers a wide range of practices which, as we have already seen, may be classified into three groups—primary, secondary and tertiary. Their specific characteristics are not of interest here except to note that they include forms of early diagnosis of certain diseases. This results in the identification and subsequent treatment of previously unrecognized disorders, some of which were included in the original schema, as well as others which are identified in the course of preventive action. This obviously results in an increase in health expenditure for the individuals concerned, at least in the short term. There is of course no way of evaluating the long-term effects of the increase in health expenditure.

One assumption we can make—an assumption which a synchronistic analysis of behaviour patterns will quite clearly demonstrate—is that if the individual comes to a proper understanding of preventive health, he will take an increased interest in his own health. His increased familiarity with and dependence on the health care system results in increased medicalization of behaviour and easier access to medical care. The medical consumption of the individual and the social groups concerned is therefore increased, since the habit of consuming medical care is culturally transmitted and related to social class.

It is also true that when people consume preventive medicine it does not have the effect of dissuading them from consuming curative medicine, nor does the former act as an alternative to the latter. On the contrary, surveys of medical consumption have shown that there is a correlation between the two which rules out any hope of economic, or at least financial advantage, from the implementation of preventive health policies. It would appear that prevention inevitably results—at least for a preliminary period which it is difficult to calculate in advance—in a paradoxical increase in health expenditure.

These findings call into question the validity of searching for and applying economic criteria only in judging the effectiveness of prevention. However it does not discredit economic and financial analysis of the mechanisms behind preventive measures and the effects anticipated, as an essential aid to making rational decisions in a field in which the moral aspect might well negate any financial constraint. Nevertheless the problem is a real one, and any attempts to contradict or deny it cannot conceal its existence.

THE ETHICS AND ECONOMICS OF PREVENTION

As I have attempted to show in this chapter, the basic ethical questions in the field of medical economics centre around the decision-making process.

The fundamental question concerns the legitimacy of basing a medical decision on economic reasoning and criteria, or given that they cannot provide a basis for decision, the relative importance we should give to them.[14] The question might be formulated as follows: what place should economic profitability occupy within the medical decision-making process? For we have in fact already left behind the question of whether or not the idea of profitability should enter into the medical field—in the current climate we cannot afford to ignore it.

However the ethical response to such a question is neither simple nor immediate. It also depends on where it arises. If, in the case of a developing country, economic logic militates against building a large technical hospital complex which would then drain off almost all the health resources of the country concerned while allowing individual medical successes, it might also call into question the allocation of funds for costly treatment for elderly persons whose life expectancy is relatively short. In both cases, the economic argument pre-empts community choice to the detriment of individual choices which do not have the same ethical value. In one case, the economic argument is reinforced, in the other it is contradicted. In any case, it does demonstrate implicitly that there is a limit to medical intervention, and that if this limit is to be accepted, it must be justified. Many people believe that since the imposition of limits does imply having to make choices, it must not be based solely on financial data. In the 1970s, faced with the danger of rationing which uncontrolled growth of health expenditures seemed certain to generate, and the reduced ability of the economic resources available to cope with such growth, many people pinned their hopes on preventive research. They believed it would result in reduction of the demand for health care and increased savings, and enable them to postpone the ethical and moral dilemmas associated with the spectre of rationing. Today, belief in this assumption is dwindling, or has at least been replaced by less mythical and more realistic reasoning. We now find ourselves confronted directly by the question of the cost of medical care and its rate of growth. It is obvious that the end purposes of medicine are not identical to those of economics. Nevertheless medicine is inextricably associated with economics, and if we do not take this into account, we might make the serious error of ignoring the economic issues altogether. For, even if medical ethics demand maximum intervention whatever the patient profile, the nature of his illness, his age, and so on, we are still dealing with limited resources and relative costs. And in economics as well as in preventive medicine, the benefit to individuals may run counter to community benefit. Choices cannot be avoided and must be clarified.

Morally speaking, we cannot let scarcity of funds engender an irrational logic of resource allocation or rationing in the health sector, with the attendant risk of waiting lists or parallel markets, and the creation of intolerable inequities. This would be unacceptable from the ethical point of view, but also from the economic point of view, since it would compromise the effectiveness of the whole system of medical intervention. The problem may seem particularly acute today, but it is by no means a new one.

It has always been necessary to make choices in allocating limited medical resources, even if these choices have previously been implicit rather than explicit. In the past they may not have been socially justified, but they tended to be accepted by the community or at least remained uncontested. Social Security systems have promoted the idea of equality of medical care, an expectation which we cannot now deny, except perhaps under special circumstances, such as war or natural disasters. The economic growth experienced by the industrialized countries has given substance to these expectations, and in a period of expansion the existence of adequate funding makes decision-making a less troublesome question. Recession makes such choices more painful and tends to reinforce the relative importance of economic criteria. However even in a recession, economic criteria must never be the sole criteria.

Economic criteria may be applied in isolation in the case of obvious wastage of resources, although we should remember that the question of the cost of health is not simply a question of wastage or bad management. The two orders of magnitude cannot be compared. In any situation where resources are limited, and in the absence of individual options, only a political decision may legitimately define the amount of resources which the community can properly allocate for health expenditures. The decision cannot be left solely to the medical profession. The basic choices must be political and democratic, and both economics and medicine must be seen as means for implementing these decisions.

REFERENCES

1. Cochrane, A. *L'inflation médicale—Réflexions sur l'efficacité de la médecine*. Paris: Galilée, 1977.
2. Israel, L. *La décision médicale*. Paris: Calmann-Lévy, 1980.
3. Levy, E., Bungener, M., Dumenil, G. and Fagnani, F. *Evaluer le coût de la maladie*. Paris: Dunod, 1977.
4. Fein, R. On measuring economic benefits of health programmes. **In**: Veatch, R., Branson, R. (eds). *Ethics and Health Policy*. Chapter 16. Cambridge Massachusetts: Ballinger Publishing Company, 1976.
5. Fuchs, V. *Who shall live?*. New York: Basic Books, 1974.
6. Leclerc, P., Majnoni, B. and Intignano, D. Interrogations sur l'efficacité de la prévention sanitaire du point de vue économique. **In**: *La Prévention Sanitaire en France*. Paris: Sirey, 1983.
7. Guillaume, H. *Le coût économique de la vie humaine*. Paris: Revue RCB, 1971.
8. Abraham, T. *Le prix de la vie humaine*. Paris: Dunod, 1972.
9. Mooney, G. H. *The Valuation of Human Life*. London: Macmillan, 1977.
10. Blomquist, G. Estimating the Value of Life and Safety: Recent Developments. **In**: *Proceedings of a Conference of the Geneva Association*. Jones-Lee, M. W. (ed). Oxford: North Holland Publishing Company, 1982.
11. Ministère de la Santé. *Pour une politique de la santé: la périnatalité*. Paris: Economie et Santé, 1972.
12. Manciaux, M. Ethique et Vaccination des Enfants. **In**: *Sciences Sociales et Santé*. Toulouse: ERES, 1984.
13. Bernard, J. Morale et Prévention des maladies. **In**: *La Prévention Sanitaire en France*. Paris: Sirey, 1983.
14. Isambert, F. A. Quelques Réflexions sur L'éthique dans le Domaine Bio-médical. **In**. *Sciences Sociales et Santé*, Toulouse: ERES, 1984.

Ethical Dilemmas in Health Promotion
Edited by S. Doxiadis

CHAPTER 11

Estimation of Occupational Risk

SIR EDWARD POCHIN

SUMMARY

A potentially important aspect of preventive medicine is reduction of risk in occupations. The difficulty lies in evaluating those risks. In comparing the magnitude of any risks to occupational health in different industries, it is necessary to find some acceptable way of evaluating the annual frequencies—for example, per 100 000 workers—of different forms of injuries and diseases. Industries differ considerably in the frequency of fatal injuries, and of non-fatal injuries causing temporary or permanent disability of different severities. There are large differences also in the frequency of fatal and non-fatal diseases attributable to working conditions or to exposure to radiation or chemicals. The relative 'weight' that should properly be attached to injuries and illnesses of different severity, and to genetic harm that may be induced by mutagenic agents, is a matter for evaluation by society as well as for any simple scientific enumeration. As an approximation to the perceived detriment of different forms of occupational harm, an 'index' of total harm is suggested which is based on the total time lost from normal health and activity as a result of non-fatal injuries or diseases, and of the time lost from a normal life expectancy as a result of injuries or diseases which cause death.

INTRODUCTION

The risks of occupational injury vary greatly in different industries, and some industries involve also a substantial risk of occupational disease. It must be an ethical imperative in preventive medicine to identify the major continuing causes for such injuries and diseases, and to ensure the greatest practicable reduction in their frequency and severity. The ethical problems involved in the acceptability of different levels of occupational risk or safety require a detailed assessment of the size of the various kinds of risk of injury or disease that are incurred in conventional occupations, and an evaluation of the amounts of risk that are likely to result from different levels of exposure to potentially harmful physical or chemical agents that may be present in the working environment. It is important therefore to review the present magnitude of different occupational risks, and the rate at which they are being reduced.

EVIDENCE ON THE FREQUENCY OF OCCUPATIONAL DAMAGE TO HEALTH

Frequency of Occupational Injuries

The frequency of occupational injuries is reported regularly in many countries for various industries, and in some cases also for industry as a whole. In different national records different criteria may be used for the inclusion of minor injuries necessitating little or no absence from work. For more severe injuries, and particularly for fatal injuries at work, however, consistent information is widely available on the frequencies of such accidents in different industries, and the rates at which these frequencies are decreasing from year to year. Specifically for fatal occupational accident rates, (the number of fatal or other accidents refer to the numbers of workers killed or injured and not to the number of accidents in which one or more were killed or injured), it is found that these rates ordinarily range from a few deaths annually per million workers at risk in the safest industries, to a few thousand such deaths per million worker-years in a few occupations as shown in Table 1.[1] When adequate and comparable, records are available over 10 or more years, these rates are in almost all cases found to be decreasing; usually by between 1 and 7 per cent of their value per year.[2]

Table 1 Fatal injury rates (annual deaths at work per 100 000 employed) in industries in the United Kingdom (average rates for years 1974–1978 except as stated).

Manufacture of clothing and footwear	0.5
Manufacture of vehicles	1.5
Manufacture of timber, furniture, etc	4.0
Manufacture of bricks, pottery, etc	6.5
Chemical and allied industries	8.5
Shipbuilding and marine engineering	10.5
Agriculture (employees)	11
Construction industries	15
Railway staff	18
Coal miners	21
Quarries	29
Non-coal miners	75
Offshore oil and gas (1967–76)	165
Deep sea fishing (accidents at sea only, 1959–68)	280

Reproduced, with permission, from a study group report to the Royal Society.[1]

Frequency of Occupational Diseases

The frequency of occupational diseases is more difficult to determine reliably. For diseases which do not cause death, there is the same difficulty in making quantitative assessments of frequency as applies to non-fatal injuries, since different industries and countries use different criteria for including sufferers in their industrial records, or for recognizing particular diseases as attributable to occupational exposures. Even with regard to fatal cases, recorded rates may be of deaths regarded as being caused by the disease, or may include deaths primarily from other causes but at which the disease was present. Moreover, additional diseases caused by environmental contaminants continue to be identified.

Two further factors make it more difficult to assess the impact of occupational diseases, and their contribution to the total risk of an industry. Firstly, a long interval, of up to several decades, may elapse between the exposure to various harmful agents such as asbestos or ionizing radiation, and the development of an induced disease. Thus, whereas the death rate from occupational injuries relates to present working conditions, that from many occupational diseases may reflect those which obtained 20 or 30 years ago.

Secondly, certain occupational diseases, such as any forms of cancer that may be induced by ionizing radiation, are indistinguishable clinically or microscopically from the much larger numbers of cancers of the same types which are likely to occur naturally. Thus while the probable numbers, for example of lung cancers in uranium miners or asbestos workers, may be assessed statistically in sufficiently large, prolonged and well-controlled epidemiological studies, the numbers arising from occupational causes in industries that have not been studied in this way can only be inferred from knowledge of the estimated risk from exposure to the harmful agents, and of the levels that applied many years previously.

The detection of an excess of tumours, and the estimation of its size, will be simpler when a normally rare malignancy is associated with exposure to a specific carcinogen, as with mesotheliomas after known exposure to asbestos or haemangiomas after exposure to vinyl chloride. For many potentially carcinogenic agents, however, no reliable risk estimate per unit dose is available from human epidemiological surveys, or from studies at low dose levels from which an excess of induced disease cannot be evaluated statistically.

EVALUATION OF TOTAL OCCUPATIONAL RISK

In the ethically important responsibility, therefore, in occupational and preventive medicine, of assessing the total risk to workers in different industries, and the rate at which these risks are being reduced, several problems need to be addressed.

1 How does the total detriment or hardship caused by non-fatal injuries compare with that from the much less common fatal injuries; and how does it compare, not only numerically, but also in its impact on the injured worker or his family?
2 For industries in which a risk of occupational disease is detectable, by what criterion could the frequency of fatal and non-fatal illnesses be compared in the detriment or hardship they entail; and can any, even approximate and tentative, comparison be proposed between the detriments resulting from injuries and diseases?
3 For industries in which a risk of occupational disease has not been detected but is to be presumed, what use of observed levels of exposure or other criteria could be suggested, to indicate whether the industry carries a high or a low total risk relative to other conventional industries in which the total risk can be observed or more directly estimated?

Little work has been done on these questions, except by use of the unduly limited criterion of the overall mortality rate, per number of worker-years at risk, from all injuries and diseases of occupational origin. No simple numerical index can define unequivocally the total risk from different kinds of detriment; and still less, the way in which different kinds of harm are regarded by different people. Yet people do make choices between alternatives which are incommensurable in any formal scientific sense; and the need to compare the safety of different industries, and particularly those involving new or unfamiliar hazards, must justify the attempt to find some acceptable index of the total harm of different working conditions.

The need for some such quantitative index of harm is most evident when an occupation necessarily involves some exposure to a potentially harmful agent, and when it cannot be assumed that there is any entirely safe level of exposure to this agent below which no harm at all will be caused. In these circumstances, it will always be important to reduce the exposure, and therefore the risk of harm, to as low a level as is practical in each industry and to establish limits of exposure which should not be exceeded in any working conditions.

Admittedly the limits set, or more exactly the average exposures which result from observance of these limits, imply the imposition of some risk, and it is here that the quantification of risk appears crucial. In principle, the presence of any avoidable occupational hazard must be ethically unacceptable. In practice, even the safest of occupations are found to involve a rather constant and quantifiable level of risk.[3] In this context, therefore, it is arguable that the control of exposures to potentially harmful chemical and physical agents should have exactly the same objective as in the control of sources of accidental injury—namely, to ensure that, whenever practical, the total risk is no greater than that achieved in the safest industries and is reduced at a comparable rate. And for this purpose, the quantification of total risk is essential.

Application to the Effects of Radiation Exposure

The problems involved, and proposals for their solution, are well illustrated by the recommendations and criteria that have been used in controlling occupational exposure to ionizing radiation (referred to from now on simply as 'radiation'). This example is worth considering in detail for a number of reasons which I will now set out.

1 No safe threshold level of radiation exposure has been established, below which some risk of harm may not occur. This may apply also to the early, and any late, effects of some chemical agents, and raises the ethical difficulties of accepting a possible risk from any exposures, however small.
2 Occupational exposure to radiation occurs in various ways and in various industries, but the measured or estimated radiation dose provides a unifying criterion of the probability of subsequent harm.
3 The effects that might result from the low doses normally occurring occupationally include different forms of cancer, of hereditarily transmitted ('genetic') defects, and perhaps also of developmental abnormalities. As may apply similarly to mutagenic chemicals, problems of aggregating different types of harm, therefore, arise within the range of diseases and induced abnormalities, as well as between the effects of diseases and of injuries.
4 The cancers, genetic defects and developmental abnormalities that might be induced by radiation are indistinguishable from similar conditions occurring naturally. Ethical problems therefore result from the impossibility of determining whether any individual disease or abnormality is induced by radiation or by 'natural' causes, except on a probabilistic basis.
5 In contrast to the situation with most chemicals, there is a substantial amount of information, from long continued human epidemiological studies, of the frequency with which cancer may be induced in different body organs, when these organs have been exposed to moderate radiation doses.[4,5] Reasonably consistent quantitative risk estimates are thus available for the carcinogenic effect of such doses.
6 In these epidemiological studies, any excess of cancers that occurs after radiation exposure needs to be distinguished statistically from the number that would have occurred naturally. The difficulty of detecting such an excess, and of estimating its size, increases rapidly as the radiation exposure, and therefore the size of the probable excess, decreases. Indeed, the size of the irradiated population that needs to be studied to detect an excess is likely to increase with the inverse square of the dose—for example, increasing 100-fold for a ten-fold reduction in dose level. The risks expected from the low annual doses involved in most occupational exposure must therefore be inferred from the frequencies observed at the much higher (50 to 500-fold higher) doses on which any reliable epidemiological findings have been based.

7 In the case of radiation, however, a large amount of radiobiological work has been done during the last 50 years on the way in which malignant, genetic and other biological effects are initiated by low or moderate doses of radiation. These studies deal quantitatively with the effects of different forms, durations and intensities of radiation exposure in causing effects at the molecular or cellular level, or in inducing genetic, malignant or developmental effects in mammals and other living forms; or in causing the relevant initial cellular damage in cultured human, as compared with other, mammalian cells.[4,5,6] The extent and quantification of such work is giving an increasingly reliable basis for inferring the risks of low doses from those observed at higher dose.

8 Finally, the development of quantitative criteria controlling occupational exposure to radiation merits particular consideration because of the longstanding and detailed international review of the nature and magnitude of radiation risks, and the way in which recommendations on sound working practice with radiation sources have been developed. International scientific commissions on radiological protection (ICRP) and on radiation units and measurements (ICRU) have operated since 1928, keeping the developing epidemiological and radiobiological information under review, and recommending criteria for measuring, monitoring and controlling radiation exposures. Moreover, in 1955 the United Nations set up a scientific committee on the effects of (atomic) radiation (UNSCEAR) to keep under surveillance and report annually on all sources of radiation exposure of populations and workers, the magnitude of doses received from these sources, the types of harmful effect that might be caused and the frequency and severity of these effects. The operation of these bodies is referred to below.

The breadth and detail of this review of radiation protection criteria could hardly have been applied to the multiplicity of potentially hazardous chemical contaminants of some working environments. Yet the way in which recommendations have been derived from valid epidemiological data on radiation effects, and translated into agreed procedures for radiation protection, seem useful to consider as a prototype for good practice in preventive medicine in other fields of occupational disease, as quantitative data on chemical and other toxicities become available.

TIME LOSS AS A BASIS FOR INTERCOMPARISON OF RISK

The first need in attempting to compare the harm caused by different forms of occupational injury, disease or disability must be to suggest some quantifiable detriment that is common to all these kinds of harm. As already mentioned, the rate of fatalities (per worker-year) is too restricted a criterion, although it may be judged to be a dominant one; and moreover, it fails to include inherited and other defects causing life-long disability. Similarly, the total number of injuries and diseases is obviously inadequate as an index of occupational risk since it is heavily influenced by the large numbers of relatively minor injuries, on which recording practices vary widely.

An aspect of harm which at least is common to all types of injury or induced disease is the length of time that is lost from full health or working capacity—or, in the extreme case of fatal injuries or diseases, lost from a normal life expectancy. Certainly any index of harm that was based on amounts of time lost in these ways would require that different 'weighting factors' should be applied to equal periods of time loss: due, for example, to being temporarily off work owing to minor injuries; to major or minor injuries causing life-long disability; to serious illnesses, and the duration and stresses involved in their cure; to prolonged or life-long disability from inherited abnormalities; or to an absolute loss of life expectancy from fatal injuries or diseases. It might be argued that the use of any criterion based on time loss was impractical because of the impossibility of determining the relative weight that should or would be given to periods of time loss due to such different types of disability. In fact, however, a necessary step in assessing the detriment that is felt to attach to different severities of injury or disease, must be to define the frequency of these forms of harm and seek an informed and considered opinion on their relative weight.

It should be useful, therefore, to examine the actual lengths of time lost from health or life resulting from accidental injuries in a range of occupations, and from recognized industrial diseases in some, including specifically the forms of harm that may be caused by occupational exposure to radiation.

TIME LOSS FROM OCCUPATIONAL INJURIES

Time Loss From Fatal Injuries

An approximate estimate of the annual loss of life expectancy from fatal injuries at work in an industry can be estimated from available records of the number of such deaths, provided that data can be obtained of the ages—or the mean age—of these deaths, and assuming that the average normal life expectancies of workers in the industry at that mean age can be taken as being equal to those of the national population.[2] Reliable estimates can usually only be made for male workers, since small numbers of fatal accidents occur in females and the ages at which such accidents occur are not often quoted.[7]

Although the mean age of accidental deaths varies somewhat in different industries, presumably because of variations in age structure of the workforce and particularly of the type of work done at different ages, the loss of life expectancy per accidental death from injury at work commonly has an average value of about 35 years in industrialized countries with normal male life expectancies at birth of 70 years or more.

Time Loss From Temporary Disabilities

In some national records, the numbers of injuries causing temporary disability are quoted, but without indicating severity or resulting time losses, except according to their involving time off work, or more than three days off work, or other general criterion. And in certain instances, the number of injuries at work which cause time off work are confounded in the record with the number of illnesses that do so, or the number of injuries incurred in travel to and from work.

In many national records, however, the annual number of injuries causing temporary disability is accompanied by figures for the mean number of days off work that each involves. When such data are available, they indicate a total time loss which is in general comparable with the losses of life expectancy from fatal accidents. It is ordinarily found, however, that in the more hazardous industries with fatal accidents of over 40 deaths per 100 000 worker-years at risk, the length of time loss from these accidents is greater than that from the non-fatal accidents, by a factor of up to 3; whereas in the safest industries with fatal accident rates less than about 5 per 100 000 worker-years (or $5.10^{-5} y^{-1}$), the time loss from the fatal accidents may be less than that from non-fatal ones, again by a factor of about 3—presumably because accidents are less likely to be fatal in the safest industries.

Even in these safer industries, however, it is likely that the detriment from fatal accidents would be considered greater than that from non-fatal ones which caused only temporary disability, if judged in terms of the time losses and the weight that would be given to them.

Time Loss From Permanent Disabilities

In principle it should be simple to estimate the length of healthy life impaired or lost as a result of injuries causing permanent disability. Records of the annual frequency of such injuries, and of the ages at which they occur, determine the total of such time loss per year of exposure of a given work-force, and so allow some measure of the risk of permanent disabilities per worker-year.

The severity of such injuries varies widely, for example, from stiffness of a finger tip to loss of two limbs. However some indication of the average level of severity can be obtained from records of the percentages of maximum pension, or disability benefit, that are awarded in the light of clinical assessments made at the time of the injury, and of subsequent re-examinations. While a majority of such awards are made at less than 30 per cent of the maximum, the total impact of such injuries—taking account both of the severity and the duration of the disabilities—seems likely to be thought of as comparable with that of fatal accidents occurring during the same period.

If so, the average value of 35 years of life lost for each accidental death should be about doubled to include the detriment from the much more frequent, but ordinarily much less severe, non-fatal accidents.

On this basis, a relatively safe light manufacturing industry with a fatal accident rate of $4.10^{-5}\,y^{-1}$—that is, with one such death occurring annually in every 25000 workers—would be regarded as having a total detriment from all occupational injuries of between two and four years lost per 1000 worker-years. A rather more hazardous industry such as mining or constructional work, with a fatality rate in the region of $20.10^{-5}\,y^{-1}$ would involve a detriment of 10 to 20 years per 1000 worker-years.

Such measures of detriment are obviously in the highest degree artificial and tentative. However, given the use of periods of life loss as at least a better criterion than fatal accident rates alone for summating different forms of harm, they do not appear to be greatly dependent on exact values of any weighting factors that might be chosen for periods of life lost in different circumstances. They could clearly be made more realistic, for example, by weighting differently the years of life lost in early or late adult life; and other developments could be suggested if their application appeared useful. Meanwhile, however, they do afford a rough basis for reviewing the relative safety or risk of occupations involving additional hazard by exposure to radiation or mutagenic chemicals, if examined according to similar estimates of harm, expressed in life or health lost through induced diseases or inherited abnormalities.

TIME LOSS FROM EFFECTS OF RADIATION EXPOSURE[2]

At present recorded levels of occupational exposure to radiation, the risks to be assessed are those of cancer induction in the exposed individual, the possibility of genetic effects in his or her progeny, and, in the case of exposure during pregnancy, effects induced in the embryo or fetus. So-called 'non-stochastic' impairments of organ function or structure, and cataract of the lens, are most unlikely except after accidents causing high exposures,[8] although impairment of lung function might possibly follow life-long exposure to high radon levels in some uranium mines.

Time Loss From Radiation-Induced Cancers

With knowledge of the annual radiation dose rate at which workers in particular occupations are exposed, estimates can be made of the probability that any cancer may develop as a result of this exposure. In most conditions, body tissues are more or less uniformly exposed, usually by external radiation, or occasionally by intake of tritium into the body. In these circumstances, the frequency of different types of cancer, and the 'latent interval' between exposure and their development, can also be estimated, on the basis of available epidemiological evidence. Or, when selective organ exposure may occur, as of the lungs in uranium miners, the probability, types and latencies of induced cancers can be assessed with reasonable confidence and accuracy.

For a given dose rate and form of exposure, therefore, it is possible to infer firstly, the types of cancer induced, and hence the numbers that are likely to prove fatal or be curable and secondly, in the case of the fatal cancers, the average resultant loss of life expectancy, given the age distribution of exposures and the latencies of the types of cancer induced. On these bases, an approximate estimate can be made of the detriment from each year's exposure of a workforce as a whole, as expressed in years of life expectancy lost (per number of worker-years at risk) from induction of fatal cancers; and the years of illness before death in the fatal cancers, and during or before treatment in those which are cured. The proportion of induced cancers which are likely to be curable can be based on the evidence that radiation-induced cancers appear to behave clinically in the same way as naturally occurring cancers of the same types, and on the long-term—that is, 15 or more years—survival of treated cancers of these types.

This obviously tentative and approximate form of assessment can be illustrated in terms of present mean levels of occupational exposure, where the average annual whole body dose rate (measured in millisieverts, mSv) of all exposed workers in the United Kingdom is 1.4,[9] and in the United States is 2.2 mSv in workers with recordable doses, or 1.1 mSv in all workers monitored for possible exposure.[10]

At an average dose rate of 2 mSv per year, the year's exposure can be estimated to result in the development of two to three fatal cancers in every 100 000 workers so exposed, with a total consequent loss of about 40 years of life expectancy (per 10^5 worker-years). To this would be added the periods of lost health and activity during the development of these cancers, and of four to five curable cancers, mainly of thyroid and skin. There is obvious difficulty in assessing the difference in suffering and disability involved in the treatment, cure and follow-up of, for example, a cancer of breast or sarcoma of bone, with severe clinical symptoms and extensive surgery or other therapy and subsequent surveillance, and the relatively minor symptoms and operative trauma usually involved in the effective cure of the types of cancer induced in skin (basal and squamous cell) and thyroid (papillary and follicular). An approximate estimate would add of the order of 10 years of severe illness and disability from all induced cancers, to the 40 years loss of life expectancy from the fatal ones induced by a year's exposure of 100 000 people at 2 mSv per year.

On these criteria, therefore, the 50 years loss of life expectancy and severe illness caused by the carcinogenic effect of present average levels of occupational exposure to radiation, would be about equal to the losses of life expectancy resulting from deaths from accidental injuries in an industry with one or two such deaths per year per 100 000 at risk, given the average loss of 35 years for each of these deaths. Or the equivalence would be to an industry with fatal accident rate of rather less than one per 10^5 worker-years, if account was taken also of the time loss from non-fatal injuries causing temporary and permanent disabilities.

In some occupations, however, dose rates are at present substantially higher (Table 2); and in the underground mining of ores of high uranium content these rates may be in the region of 25 mSv per year (effective dose equivalent), if account is taken of inhaled radon and thoron daughter products and dusts, and of external radiation from the surrounding rock. In such cases, the carcinogenic risk could be expressed as a time loss of about 600 years per 10^5 worker-years, or equivalent to the total injury risk of an industry with about 10 such deaths per 10^5 worker-years; or substantially less than the fatal accident rate in deep uranium mining itself, which may exceed $30.10^{-5}\,y^{-1}$.

Table 2 United Kingdom rates of occupational exposure.

Occupation		$mSv\,y^{-1}$ Effective dose equivalent
By results of monitoring		
Nuclear Fuel Cycle		
Fuel fabrication	1983	1.3
Fuel enrichment	1983	0.4
Fuel reprocessing	1983	7.0
Power stations	1982	1.4
Research		
Nuclear	1983	2.8
Universities	1980	0.1
Industry		
Radiographers	1982	1.7
Tritium workers	1980	3.4
Radionuclide supply	1982	3.8
Other industrial	1982	0.4
Medical		
Diagnostic staff	1981	0.4
Radiotherapy staff	1981	2.6
Radionuclide work	1981	0.3
By estimates of enhanced natural exposure		
Coal miners		1.2
Non-coal miners		26.0
Air crews		1.6
Average, all occupationally exposed		1.4

Source: Hughes, J. S. and Roberts, G. C. *The radiation exposure of the UK population — 1984 review*. National Radiological Protection Board report NRPB-R173. NRPB, Chilton, Oxon. 1984.[9] Reproduced with permission of the National Radiological Protection Board.

It may be noted that these estimates of carcinogenic risk are based on an 'absolute risk' hypothesis, with a probability of 1.25×10^{-5} mSv^{-1} of fatal cancer induction.[11] The so-called 'relative risk' hypothesis postulates for most cancers a subsequent increase of cancers after radiation which is proportional to the natural cancer rate at the corresponding ages.[5] This hypothesis predicts a number of induced cancers which is about 1.6 times that predicted by the absolute risk hypothesis, after doses received regularly throughout working life. Since the relative risk causes the greatest increases during later life, however, when the natural incidence is greatest, the mean loss of life expectancy per cancer is less than on the absolute risk hypothesis, and the total life loss is also rather less.[2]

Time Loss From Radiation-Induced Genetic Defects

The probability that genetic effects will be caused by occupational exposure depends upon the exposures received before the conception of children. The magnitude of this probability therefore depends rather critically upon the age and sex structure of the working population, and the age at which exposure starts, since the mean age at conception of her children in women is typically about 26 years, and about 31 years in men (mothers, 25.9 ± 1.7 SD years; fathers 30.6 ± 2.9 SD years in 41 countries.[12])

The probability of a genetic defect, of greater or less severity, induced per unit dose received before conception of a child has been assessed by the UN Radiation Committee, UNSCEAR. The Committee assesses the number of various types of defect that are liable to be expressed in the first generation after exposure, and in all generations at equilibrium after continuing exposure.[13] These estimates are necessarily based on the rates of mutation and of chromosomal aberrations observed in mice, in other primates, and in human cells observed *in vitro*, in the absence of any genetic effects that can be detected in large human populations that have been exposed to radiation.

The members of the Committee with experience in human genetics have also published an assessment, which is valuable in respect of time loss criteria, of the impact of the various types and frequencies of genetic defect induced by radiation. Thus, for each of these main types of defect, they have recorded the years of life, if any, before any impairment develops, the years of any substantial impairment, and the average years of life expectancy lost by premature death in those inheriting the defect.

It is therefore possible, by combining the frequency with which defects are likely to be induced, with the length of impaired and lost life which they cause, to derive a figure for years lost which can be compared with the years lost through carcinogenic effects. Here it is necessary to specify the starting age of exposure, and to estimate separately for the two sexes in view of the earlier mean age at conception of children in women. In a working population of women exposed at 2 mSv per year from age 20 to 65 years, the average annual contribution to the genetic detriment expressed in all subsequent generations would be equivalent to 17 years per 10^5 worker-years. In men, with their later mean age at conceptions, the figure would be about 29 years. The difference between numbers of effects in men or women may be rather greater in view of evidence of a greater induction rate of genetic effects in male than in female germ cells.[13]

These figures compare with the average estimate of 50 years (per 10^5 worker-years) from carcinogenesis: or, more exactly, with 63 years in women and 37 years in men, because of differences in cancer induction in the two sexes (particularly of breast cancer, and to a lesser extent of thyroid cancer).

Time Loss From Radiation Effects on the Conceptus

Different kinds of effect may be caused in the developing child by exposures occurring at different stages in its development. During critical periods while the individual organs and body structures are developing, malformations may occur causing subsequent defects in the function of the organ including that of the nervous system. Failure of the fertilized ovum to implant in the uterine wall may result from exposure, with death of the conceptus, during the earliest days after its fertilization. Damage to the germ cells may result in inherited abnormalities in subsequent generations. And there is evidence that exposures during development in utero, as in later life, are associated with an increased cancer rate subsequently, the induction rate per unit dose being perhaps twice that in adults.

The frequency with which pregnancies occur in full-time workers will vary, and exposures may continue during pregnancy only at reduced rates. Estimates of harm can, however, be made under the somewhat maximizing assumptions that pregnancies occur at the same rates as in the whole population, and that exposures continue without reduction during the whole of all pregnancies. The doses delivered to the conceptus throughout the pregnancy, or in the relevant critical periods during which different harmful effects may be induced, can then be combined with estimates of the risk of these effects per unit dose delivered.

Taking account of the impairments and losses of life expectancy for each of the effects induced in the fetus, an estimate is obtained in terms of life loss occurring during any pregnancy, and hence per year of work with a normal frequency of pregnancies. Under these assumptions, and with exposure continuing unchanged throughout the whole of all pregnancies, the equivalent years of detriment, per year of exposure at 2 mSv per year in a workforce of 100 000 women, would be of about 100 years, about half of this total being from developmental defects—if induced without threshold[14]—with lesser contributions from non-implantation of the fertilized ovum and from induction of fatal cancers, and minor components from induced genetic effects and from curable cancers.[2]

SUMMATION OF RISKS OF DIFFERENT KINDS

Any numerical summation of different kinds of occupational risk will inevitably be crude and in some respects unrealistic; and the use of time loss as a unifying factor in comparing different risks has obvious inadequacies. The present discussion of the effects of industrial injury and of radiation exposure can only serve as an illustration of an approach to this problem, and of the questions which require answers from society in making such an attempt.

Given that it must be irresponsible, however, to allow working conditions without making any assessment of the risk that they involve, some criterion must surely be adopted—and the most realistic criterion that is available—to compare the total risks of different occupations, and, in particular, those involving predictable risks of induced disease or abnormality. It is obviously inadequate to wait for evidence from retrospective surveys of the frequency of such diseases if, as in the case of ionizing radiation, the abnormalities are only likely to be expressed decades or generations after the causative exposures, to be individually indistinguishable from naturally occurring abnormalities of the same type, and only to be detectable with difficulty statistically following the present low rates of occupational radiation exposure.

In this sense the present review, however incomplete, could serve as a discussion document in the necessary process of developing opinion on valid methods of aggregating risks, and on the weight that is felt to apply to different types of risk.

The assessment of the effects of radiation exposure offers a useful example of an approach that should, in principle, apply similarly to a predictive risk assessment for various chemical and other mutagenic agents that may be present in the working environment. Here, the process of review is informative, both as regards the establishment of national regulations and the development of a concept of acceptable risk.

The purely scientific data base is strong—the 1982 report of the UN Radiation Committee alone contains some 770 pages and 3600 literature references,[13] and is required reading in any field of radiation protection. The International Commission on Radiological Protection publishes reports of its recommendations, of the work of its standing committees, and of scientific task groups set up to review particular fields of radiation protection. Reports are thus issued from meetings of 70 to 80 scientists of a wide range of relevant disciplines and from some 20 nations, with participation by the World Health Organization, the International Atomic Energy Agency, the International Labour Organization, the Secretariat of UNSCEAR, and other United Nations bodies.

The Commission's reports are, very properly, in the form of recommendations since it must be a national responsibility to decide on the standards of safety that are to be maintained in its industries. The recommendations are of the dose limits and procedures, the observance of which would ensure that average exposures involve only a low—and quantitatively specified—risk.

These recommendations are very widely adopted. It would, however, be understandable if some country considered that its national urgencies justified rather greater risks than were recommended as optimal; or if others were able to apply the Commission's recommendation, that 'all exposures should be kept as low as reasonably achievable . . . '[11] with considerable stringency.

An important step is therefore involved in the various national mechanisms for review of international recommendations in the light of the levels of safety or risk that they would achieve: a review both by scientific bodies of their validity, and by bodies with broader reference for their impact on and acceptance by society. Thus in the case of the European Community, this review is undertaken both by a scientific committee and by the Economic and Social Committee.

Within the nation, the same recommendation, as quoted in full, that 'exposures should be kept as low as reasonably achievable, economic and social factors being taken into account', can provide the essential ground for interaction between government inspectorates and individual industrial practices. The words reflect the likelihood that increased national expenditure on protective measures would result in lower exposures, but that there will be some point beyond which further expenditure would be better used for other purposes of the protection of human health and welfare.

If such interactions are developed in the light of both actual levels of risk and levels of risk perceived by society, we can hope to progress towards a better perspective than at present on what levels of safety, and rates of risk reduction, can be achieved; and even on how low a level of risk might properly be regarded as 'acceptable' in different circumstances of industrial exposure in which some amount of risk is always present. These are considerations of obvious and substantial ethical importance to the community on which it is necessary that society should develop a clear and informed opinion. Such an opinion, however, requires that not only the types, but also the magnitudes, of different occupational risks should be taken into account. As a necessary contribution to such a review, a method of estimating and comparing the magnitude of total occupational risks is needed. The proper formulation of an appropriate index of occupational harm requires urgent consideration in consequence.

REFERENCES

1. *Risk Assessment: Report of a Study Group*. London: Royal Society, 1983.
2. Quantitative bases for developing an unified index of harm. A report to the International Commission on Radiological Protection. *Annals of the ICRP* **15** (3) 1–64, 1985. Oxford: Pergamon Press.
3. Pochin, E. E. Occupational and other fatality rates. *Community Health* 1974, **6**: 2–13.
4. *Sources and effects of ionising radiation*. United Nations Scientific Committee on the Effects of Atomic Radiation, 1977 report to the General Assembly. New York: United Nations, 1977.

5. *The effect on populations of exposure to low levels of ionising radiation*. Committee on the biological effects of ionising radiation (BEIR III report). Washington DC: National Academy Press, 1980.
6. Boice, J. D. and Fraumeni, J. F. (eds). *Radiation Carcinogenesis: Epidemiology and Biological Significance*. New York: Raven Press, 1984.
7. Schaaf, E. and Hennig, J. *Berufsspezifische Unfallrisiken zum Vergleich mit Risiken durch berufsbedingte Strahlenbelastung*. Bericht Nr. St. Sch. 905. Köln: Bundesministers des Innern, 1984.
8. Non-stochastic effects of ionising radiation, ICRP Publication 41. *Annals of the ICRP* **14**, 1984.
9. Hughes, J. S. and Roberts, G. C. *The radiation exposure of the UK population—1984 review*. National Radiological Protection Board report NRPB-R173. Chilton, Oxon: NRPB, 1984.
10. Kumazawa, S., Nelson, D. R. and Richardson, A. C. B. *Occupational exposure to ionising radiation in the United States*. Washington, DC: US Environmental Protection Agency, 1984.
11. Recommendations of the International Commission on Radiological Protection. ICRP Publication 26. *Annals of the ICRP* **1**, 1977.
12. *Demographic Handbook 1981*. New York: United Nations, 1983.
13. *Ionising radiation*: *Sources and Biological Effects*. United Nations Scientific Committee on the Effects of Atomic Radiation, 1982 report to the General Assembly. New York: United Nations, 1982.
14. Otake, M. and Schull, W. J. In utero exposure to A-bomb radiation and mental retardation: a reassessment. *Br J Radiol* 1984; **57**: 409–414.

PART C
SPECIFIC ISSUES

Ethical Dilemmas in Health Promotion
Edited by S. Doxiadis

CHAPTER 12

Ethical Aspects of Reproductive Medicine

HELEEN M. DUPUIS

SUMMARY

This chapter provides a survey of the various moral implications of reproduction technology as far as matters of prevention and public health are concerned. In particular, it raises ethical questions and problems related to individual autonomy and the paternalism of the public authority or the state. It concentrates on the particular areas of population control, fertility and infertility, the allocation of resources in reproductive technology, the protection of the embryo and the quality of progeny.

INTRODUCTION

The many medical methods of controlling procreation now available raise numerous practical questions. Some of these concern *quantity* of procreation. Quantity is perhaps usually viewed in a negative sense where birth control has been made possible by contraception, sterilization and abortion. Quantity can also be viewed in a positive sense where an increase in births has resulted from advances in knowledge about undesired sterility. Conception can now be achieved by various means including hormonal stimulation, *in vitro* fertilization (IVF), and artificial insemination by donor (AID).

In addition, more and more attention is being paid to the *quality* of progeny. The techniques of early detection of fetal defects, an increasing insight into hereditary diseases, together with selective or eugenic abortion, increase the possibility of manipulating outcome. These advances in the field of manipulation of human fertility, however, raise important ethical questions. One of the most urgent and intractable of these is 'who will decide?'

It is of course obvious that the individual couples concerned are the first to decide on the quantity and quality of their offspring, and in the normal course of events there is no outside agency involved beyond the normal prenatal and obstetric care. But when any complications or difficulties arise, more people necessarily become involved—the child that is either born or not, the physician and other medical and paramedical personnel, the government or State and finally also society at large who may be said to have an interest in the size of population growth and in the health and wellbeing of children born. And it is in this context that the 'who will decide' question must be examined.

In this chapter I propose, therefore, to concentrate on this crucial relationship between individual wishes and the common good, represented by the government or state and society. What can and should be left to the personal choice of the individual couple? It is a basic ethical question which arises in every area of medical ethics. It is perhaps particularly relevant in the present context of reproduction ethics.

POPULATION CONTROL

There have been efforts by governments in various countries to introduce population control policies but these have not been very successful. Birth control is a most personal matter and it is difficult to influence unless a government is prepared to interfere with individual liberty to what would seem to most of us to be an unacceptable extent. The population control measures in China, described by Einsenberg in Chapter 9, are one example of this.

Many factors seem to define the size of a family and nearly all of them are difficult to manage or manipulate.[1] It would seem, therefore, that in a society which respects the rights of its citizens, a strict population policy is virtually impossible. Guidance, the availability of effective contraceptives, financial incentives will probably have only marginal significance. No Western country appears able to get beyond a limited change of attitude although a number undoubtedly feel the need to exercise some control. So is government allowed to influence people, on the strength of what arguments, and to what extent? The fundamental principle of the autonomy of the citizen is highly valued in most Western countries. And if it concerns a vision of our private lives, of sexuality, marriage and parenthood, this autonomy appears inviolable.

But those who look further will see that this autonomy, if present at all, is quite recent and certainly not absolute in character. On the contrary, many societies have awarded themselves the right to ban the unrestricted sale of contraceptives, and on matters such as divorce, abortion, and homosexuality, the rules are sometimes very strict. This kind of restriction of individual freedom is often upheld on the strength of religious arguments whose precise justification is vague. From a moral point of view, an ethical justification means a rational answer to the question of how a particular restriction of individual freedom can be defended. The only acceptable answer seems to be that stronger interests of individuals are involved since, in the end, any ethical justification amounts to the question whether and to what extent an action serves the interest of the people.

PATERNALISM AND AUTONOMY: ASSESSMENT OF THE INTEREST OF INDIVIDUALS

This takes us to the central issue—discussed also in detail in Chapter 7—the relationship between paternalism of the state and the autonomy of the individual. Who determines what is in the interest of the individual citizen—the citizen himself or the community? And how far should individual autonomy go? Is the government allowed to set limits and, if so, to what extent?

I should like to defend the thesis that an infringement—by the state—of the individual autonomy can be defended subject to the following conditions: (1) the integrity of the human body should never under any circumstances be violated; (2) the curtailment of freedom should be in the interests of the people concerned; (3) restriction of liberty should also be for the furtherance of the common good.

We now face another problem—is it possible to state what is in general harmful to or in the interest of people, both individuals (condition 2) and the society at large (condition 3)? If the essence of autonomy is that the individuals themselves determine their own interests, then paternalism means that others do this for them.[2] This question of paternalism versus antipaternalism is also discussed fully by Beauchamp in Chapter 7 of this book.

It may be true that what others regard as being in someone's interest, is also perceived as such by the individual concerned. An example of this is the classic doctor-patient relationship, in which it is usually taken for granted that what the doctor thinks best for the patient, is in fact best for him. In other words, agreement is already there and consequently the question 'who will decide?' need not be asked. Autonomy and paternalism become compatible.

While we cannot take it for granted that one person can decide what is good for another, it is a fact that in many situations people decide about each other's interest. A person who is seriously injured, for example, should be taken immediately to hospital; if at all possible we save someone who is in danger of being drowned; and we pull away a child that stretches out its hand to a vicious dog. The question is now whether there are situations in which the interest of a person is so self-evident, that the government is allowed and able to determine this for him. Implicitly we then take the view that the person concerned, after proper consideration and having the same information, would reach the same conclusion. On the basis of the interest of a person with a hazardous life-style, for example, it can be defended that the government takes measures to prevent illness or injury. This might imply a restriction of freedom. So the values of the freedom of the individual, his health, and possibly the common good have to be balanced against each other. Such a rational consideration might well result in compulsory vaccination but also in the obligation to wear safety-belts while motoring. It is clear here that a slight infringement of personal rights is advantageous both to the person concerned and to society which has an interest in averting an epidemic of infectious disease or in preventing injury from road accidents.

IS POPULATION CONTROL MORALLY JUSTIFIABLE?

Is it possible, then, to defend a population policy on the strength of the above line of reasoning? In my view the first condition, concerning the integrity of the body, excludes the use of any means other than persuasion. Compulsory contraception, let alone compulsory abortion or sterilization, cannot be morally defended, nor can society compel a woman to bear children. Questions also arise about the interest of the couple concerned and the interest of society, the second and third conditions. It is unlikely that we would be able to determine, within reasonable limits, how large or small a population should be. The same may be true for family size although there is some evidence of a relationship between size of family and the health of mother and children.[3,4] We could argue that it can never be in the interests of a family itself to have numerous offspring and that a very large family makes a prolonged claim on resources as a result of which smaller families might suffer. This may justify pressure by public authority for a limitation on size of family. It seems, however, that an adequate population policy is hard, if not impossible, to achieve if we continue to consider the integrity of the body as a matter of the greatest importance. Nor can we satisfy the other conditions regarding the interests of individuals and the common good. Thus government can do little but offer good and effective guidance although the opportunities for doing this are limited since family planning has its own rationale. Furthermore we may wonder whether the argument of individual autonomy does not imply the possibility that the individual knows how to handle manipulating information. The risk of real manipulation of family planning by means of information seems small, and in practice this appears to be the case. A far more important incentive is the easy availability of contraceptives.

FERTILITY AND INFERTILITY: AN INDIVIDUAL AND SOCIAL PROBLEM

Population control has only become an issue because of the availability of contraception in many countries. At the individual level, the use of contraception can raise a number of problems, including in some cases what should be the attitude and involvement of government. Is government, for example, permitted to promote the use of the condom to prevent the sexually transmitted diseases that are almost endemic in some countries? AIDS, gonorrhea and chlamydia are serious health hazards which could be limited by the use of condoms.

Abortion

Contraception and abortion for other than medical reasons are sometimes regarded as practically synonymous and there are countries where abortion does play an important role in population control. Nobody, however, would consider this to be a satisfactory state of affairs firstly because of the possible implications for the woman concerned. Secondly, there is also a growing awareness of the rights of the embryo (defined in the usual sense of a pregnancy duration of less than two months) or fetus (pregnancy more than two months) which is terminated by abortion. Is it the task of government to protect the embryo against its mother? Society has no generally accepted view on this—one community may hold a completely different view from another. Nor is there any moral consensus about fetal protection or the role of government in this context but many questions arise.

Does the right to the integrity of the human body mean that a woman can be compelled to complete her pregnancy? Is the embryo entitled to his mother's body? In some cases the inclination will obviously be to answer 'no' to both these questions. In most countries, for example, pregnancy as a result of rape is an acceptable reason for abortion. But from the point of view of the fetus it is of little importance whether it came into being as a result of a loving embrace or of an act of violence. What then are the rights of the embryo or fetus and how consistently should a government protect these? The same dilemma also arises with a technique like *in vitro* fertilization (IVF) and with experiments on fetal material.

Sterilization

The most effective method of preventing pregnancy—sterilization—presents fewer problems. Yet here too the question of the role of government arises. Do individuals have a free choice about sterilization, should the government have a say in the matter, or should it be left to the professional group—the physicians? It may seem unlikely that anyone can be in a better position to judge the issue than the individual requesting sterilization. But from a preventive point of view, there are hazards. A decision taken rashly or emotionally, may be regretted, circumstances may change, and reversal of sterilization may be unsuccessful or impossible.

Analysis of the following example illustrates some of the extremely complex issues that can arise in this area. A woman with three children underwent sterilization. She subsequently divorced, met another man and requested that the sterilization be reversed. This proved impossible. *In vitro* fertilization was carried out and resulted in a multiple pregnancy. This was not acceptable to her and so a partial abortion to retain one or two fetuses was considered.

The first step in this case seems simple—a woman with a complete family is sterilized, a simple affair in a country without predominant religious objections to the practice. Then a divorce takes place. A relationship with another man is formed and the new couple want to have a child. This is impossible because of the earlier decision in favour of sterilization. Then a mechanism which is becoming increasingly common comes into operation: circumstances have changed, a previous decision becomes unacceptable, and if something can be done to alter it (that is, if a technique is available), it must be done at any price. The same mechanism operates also for the multiple pregnancy that is achieved by IVF.

Perhaps we should question this whole procedure and ask whether an individual should be permitted to adopt such an attitude in her own and society's interests, and whether it is possible to defend such claims on our general resources.

Here a new argument emerges—namely, that of the allocation of scarce resources. From the point of view of distributive justice, there may be a role here for government unless we simply accept the principle of first come first served. Finally, there is the interest of the fetuses destroyed in the partial abortion. Is it, under all these circumstances, still possible to justify such a course of action?

PREVENTION AND THE ALLOCATION OF SCARCE RESOURCES

As is the case throughout the field of health care, allocation of resources is relevant and important, and it is perhaps even more important in the field of reproduction than in the case of operations which are strictly therapeutic in character.

Can we, for example, justify a decision to try to reverse a sterilization operation on a woman with three healthy children who underwent sterilization at her own request. When the reversal is unsuccessful, is it justifiable to offer the very specialized technique of *in vitro* fertilization? When that technique is successful but produces an unacceptable result from the patient's point of view, in the form of a multiple pregnancy, is it justifiable to offer an even more specialized technique, selective abortion, to try to rectify the situation? In short how many demands on limited resources can we allow one individual to make at the expense of alternative uses of these resources?

Individual Autonomy and Priorities in Health Care

The term allocation of scarce resources implies that it is not possible for everyone to get what he asks for, and it is sometimes argued that this will lead to an undesirable limitation of the right to self-determination or autonomy. But does it? First and foremost, autonomy, or rather the right of self-determination, has to do with the integrity of the body, the person and his privacy, and it implies that infringements of these need not be tolerated. For health care this implies particularly the right to refuse medical treatment. In many Western countries this right has been acknowledged.

The second aspect of self-determination has also gained wide acceptance but remains less strong than the first one—this is a case of self-determination in the sense of self-manipulation. The question that arises is whether the individual is allowed to do with his body as he pleases. The answer to this typically ethical question is often determined and thus restricted by religious considerations. But there is another fundamental restriction—with most kinds of self-manipulation another person is needed, namely a physician, who can cooperate or refuse to take the action requested. Especially interesting in the context of autonomy is the position of the physician who refuses to act as the patient wishes. Will society allow him this freedom, or will he be obliged to do what patients want?

Finally—and this is pre-eminently a case belonging to public health—self-determination of the individual may be regarded as the right to claim certain provisions. The limit set to this is in the first place economic in character. But this economic limit is a moral limit at the same time: things that are required and received by one person, cannot be offered to others. The question of a fair distribution of resources is also implied by this third aspect of self-determination.

PROTECTION OF THE EMBRYO: A MATTER OF PUBLIC AUTHORITY

New perinatal technology enables people who formerly would have remained childless, to become parents. This is not only true for women who are sterile, but also for women without husbands, for lesbian couples, and even for homosexual male pairs. It is almost certain that the *in vitro* fertilization technique in particular, in combination with artificial insemination by donor, will be an attractive possibility in the future for those who do not wish to have sexual intercourse, but nevertheless want to be parents.

I do not propose to discuss all the moral aspects of these new possibilities, but will confine my remarks to those with possible consequences for public authority or public health in general. Several issues then, should be considered. First of all, there is the important matter of *prevention*. This pertains especially to certain types of female sterility, caused sometimes by previously contracted sexually transmitted diseases. Thus if we have available a morally questionable technology, as IVF is said by some to be, which can get round this problem, we should first of all be aware of the possibility of preventing the types of sterility involved. This prevention can only be carried out through adequate information freely and fully available to those concerned: any form of constraint in matters such as the choice of methods of contraception is not possible. But there is certainly no reason to withhold information: it is clearly both in the interest of the women themselves and of society to restrict sexually transmitted diseases.

Apart from prevention, there remains the question of the use of the IVF technology, combined, in some cases, with AID. The most difficult moral question appears to be the status of the embryo, especially of the so-called 'leftovers' and their cryopreservation. Secondly there are questions that follow from special uses of this technique such as, surrogate motherhood, for example. Thirdly we have to face problems surrounding selection of patients which brings us back again to the allocation of resources.

Status of the Embryo

The IVF technology implies the assumption that very early human life—that is embryos which are only a few days old—are in fact disposable. In societies where abortion is permitted, it has been decided that embryos have no rights of their own; their lives depend on the will of their mothers. But if embryos (or fetuses) have to lose their lives, it should be for strong reasons—namely, an emergency situation in their mother's life. *In vitro* fertilization, however, takes it for granted that embryos—when they are not yet implanted in the womb—are things that can be used or disposed of, not in emergencies, but by definition. I do not think this can lead to an ultimate argument against IVF. But it should encourage us towards a certain caution when considering the IVF technology.

Another problem, raised by IVF, concerns the theoretical possibilities of having one's own children borne by another person. Should a government allow such a practice? Public opinions differ on the matter. But one thing is certain—the vision and the laws of parenthood will have to be revised if we accept surrogate motherhood. Here again we should define the limits of the intervention of government. Let us assume that we have convincing arguments against surrogate motherhood, for instance because there is evidence that the pregnancy can result in psychological trauma for the surrogate mother. Should we then ask for it to be legally prohibited? Or is it for the people to decide for themselves? Looking at the criteria mentioned before, I do not think the arguments in favour of a general prohibition are sufficient. The question as to whether surrogate motherhood could cause damage to society or to the common good remains to be decided, and the whole subject requires to be examined much more fully.

QUALITY OF PROGENY

One last issue remains to be discussed. It is quite different from the previous ones and has not yet been mentioned—the quality of life of future children. Perinatal technology enables us to detect congenital disease or handicap in the fetus. Two harassing questions result from this advanced technology: which handicaps are compatible with a life worthy of a human being, and who shall decide?

In the prevention of diseases antenatal diagnosis plays an important role. Such diagnosis is almost always requested by the pregnant woman, and usually, if something seriously wrong is found, an abortion is performed. There is certainly no obligation for a woman to undergo such an examination nor submit herself or her baby to an abortion. Indeed the right to integrity of the body forbids such an obligation.

Nevertheless, from the point of view of the child, the family, society, and even the woman herself, in some cases one could rightly ask if their interests are served by a prolongation of the pregnancy. Already law suits for 'wrongful life' have taken place in some countries. From a moral point of view, the arguments for abortion may be strong but they can never be strong enough to infringe on the right of the pregnant woman to decide about herself and her child. Even if she makes what is obviously the wrong choice, we can do no more than hope that she will not regret it later—there are no ways to compel her to take one decision rather than another. Another question is whether this remains true in the case of a mentally handicapped girl who becomes pregnant and is at risk for the birth of a handicapped child? I am not sure about her rights to a decision of her own, although it seems unthinkable that she should be obliged to have an abortion if she herself does not want to. But if, as is the case in some countries, an enforced sterilization of mentally handicapped persons is considered morally acceptable, should not we consider enforced abortion also?

We do not have an answer to these urgent and uncomfortable questions but they must be acknowledged and examined. The ultimate answer may be that human beings should treat each other as human beings—from this starting point we can find the limits of our moral standards, both on an individual level and on the level of society.

REFERENCES

1. Hardin, G. The tragedy of the commons. *Science* 1968; **162**: 1243–1248.
2. Beauchamp, T. L. and Childress, J. F. *Principles of Biomedical Ethics*. New York, Oxford: Oxford University Press, 1983; 59–66.
3. Wray, J. D. *Population Pressure on Families: Family Size and Child Spacing. Reports on Population/Family Planning*. New York: The Population Council, 1971.
4. *Statistical Indices of Family Health*. Report of a WHO Study Group. Technical Report Series 587. Geneva: WHO, 1976.

Ethical Dilemmas in Health Promotion
Edited by S. Doxiadis

CHAPTER 13

Promotion of Child Health

M. MANCIAUX AND E. A. SAND

SUMMARY

In many fields of child health, whether curative or preventive in nature, new ethical issues arise since it is often impossible to extrapolate data from adult populations and situations. The main considerations of this chapter concern the physical and mental health of children and screening procedures. We also cover more specific problems such as child abuse and neglect, school failure, psychosocial and mental retardation and so on. Emphasis is also put on confidentiality in paediatric practice, on competence to consent, on research and training and the related ethical aspects of all these. The chapter ends by highlighting the main obstacles and constraints which make it difficult to apply these principles in practice.

INTRODUCTION

It is our intention in this chapter to review some of the ethical problems that arise in daily paediatric practice, especially in relation to preventive activities. We shall then try to relate these problems to the general rules governing medical ethics and to pinpoint many obstacles and constraints which make it difficult to apply these principles in practice. Finally we will discuss some aspects of training and research.

PRACTICAL PROBLEMS

Many burning ethical problems arise in a paediatric practice. The specialty tends to be more curative than preventive in nature but some of the ethical problems have nevertheless preventive implications. This is so in the case of induced abortion, for example, when it is used to prevent congenital abnormalities; and in neonatal resuscitation and its withdrawal in order to avoid subsequent handicap.

In research, trials involving children are also necessary since it is impossible simply to extrapolate to children results obtained from adults.

Physical Health and Ethics

In the somatic field, *immunizations* represent a model, both for experimental trials (the last step in clinical experiment of most vaccines has to involve young children) and for their use in daily practice.[1] The problem is more simple for those vaccines which confer only an individual immunity, like tetanus toxoid (except the mother-fetus passive transmission). On the other hand, most vaccines are also useful through the herd immunity mechanism: it is then necessary to immunize a large portion of the community according to the objective of the programme—control, elimination, or eradication. The ethical issues vary accordingly. In this field, public opinion should be clearly and objectively informed in order to be able to give a valid consent. This is especially important in those countries where immunization is organized on a voluntary basis. However, some conflict can arise between health professionals and the media, the latter being not bound by ethical obligations concerning the scientific validity of the information they publish. Everybody remembers what happened in the United Kingdom where the dissemination of misleading information on the possible complications of whooping cough vaccine has led to a considerable decrease of the acceptance of immunizations. The reappearance or, at least, an increasing incidence of a communicable disease preventable by immunization exceeded by far the risks of side-effects of this specific vaccination. Such a harmful situation should be avoided by better coordination between doctors, health administrators and media specialists, at least those who take an ethical approach in their professional responsibility.[1]

More recently developed *screening procedures* tend to expand—both in population coverage and the number of screened conditions—and to be better scrutinized on their cost-benefit and ethical aspects.

In the field of prenatal *screening for congenital abnormalities*, no general rule can be defined since national policies are quite different as regards, for instance, the availability of induced abortion in the case of congenital defects so detected. Yet it must be recalled that the crucial debate is whether the condition constitutes a serious harm and whether the medical profession representing society has anything to offer in order to alleviate the burden.

For screening procedures in the neonatal period, as for those later in life, a first question arises: are we sure that the screening process will not be harmful to the subjects? Not so long ago, before the second world war, in some European countries, schoolchildren underwent a radioscopic examination each year. We know now that such screening procedures may not be innocuous.

Screening for mental deficiency by using a tool like the intelligence quotient or IQ—so rightly criticized as being culture-bound—has led in many countries to the incorrect identification of a huge number of children who are not mentally deficient but only culturally disadvantaged.[2] The importance that parents and school teachers may attach to the results of this testing is disproportionate to its limited value. It is therefore essential to consider not only the cost of such extensive surveys but also the potential harmful effects on the attitudes of the adults towards the children with low scores. Even more harmful may be such testing and the divulging of the results to the self-esteem of the children themselves.

A second important question is how serious is the problem one wants to screen for? This does not involve only the prevalence of the condition, but its duration and level of harmfulness, as well as the existing possibilities for treatment and cure. A cost–benefit evaluation is necessary which, in the case of phenylketonuria, for instance, would lead to a positive answer, at least in developed countries. The process may produce only 10 cases per year in a country like Belgium, but the test is cheap and routinely performed, and the condition can be alleviated. However, the same evaluative approach could lead to an opposite decision for a developing country where other conditions deserve priority.

In this context another problem arises. Mass screening or examination of children for any condition, be it mental inferiority, biochemical errors, signs of malnutrition, may be understood by the parents as leading inevitably to the prevention of such diseases or handicaps. This is, however, not always so. We have therefore to consider the 'ethics of false hope' and to explain what the children and their families are likely to gain from the screening project. If we fail to be quite clear on this point we break the ethical rule of absolute sincerity towards the subjects of our investigations. But we also lose the confidence of the parents and the community in general if they expect more than the project can offer. Any future request for cooperation and consent will then be met with mistrust.

Child Abuse and Neglect

Just at the border between physical and mental health, child abuse and neglect—perhaps the most touchy and difficult issue in modern social paediatrics—many controversial ethical considerations originate.

At what level of risk should one take care of the family and the child and possibly provoke a separation of the child, for its own safety? In some cases where this has not been done, the child has died. On the other hand, most families fear and resent separation, and if one separates the child from its family, it can be very difficult to begin the serious medical and psychological help needed by the family itself.

The dialogue between family and health professionals represents another intractable problem—how to prevent the occurrence of child abuse, or maltreatment? What is the normal acceptable level of aggressive behaviour in parents?[3] For certain families in some social groups, aggression in the form of physical punishment does not have the same meaning as it might have in other family settings. If we are attempting to help a child and family and we start by giving a normative statement about the harm aggression can do, we risk cutting the channels of communication and jeopardizing any possibility of real help.

In Brussels, and in several other European cities, new ways of taking care of these children and families are currently being applied. They can be described as primary prevention after establishing a very early diagnosis of high risk mothers during pregnancy. The mothers are involved in a psychological or psychotherapeutic dialogue about their pregnancy and the developing child. The psychologist helps the mother to express, define and clarify her own difficulties, which enables her to overcome them, or some of them, and to reinforce her general abilities to cope with difficult life situations.[4] This approach, when successful, respects the physical and mental health of the child and preserves the integrity and the autonomy of the family.

Child Mental Health and Ethics

Problems of mental health have a high prevalence in children and can reach 12 to 15 per cent of the child population in some countries if one includes neurotic manifestations, mental retardation, low IQ and other conditions such as child psychosis. Mental health has many aspects. Mental health troubles are manifold. Problems in mental health, even more than those in physical health are multivariate in character and it is often difficult to point out potential causal associations. Moreover such statistical associations are the main prerequisite of any preventive intervention.

School maladjustment or failure can affect as many as 40 to 50 per cent of all children in some European countries.[5] In this area too, prevention and early intervention may be more efficient than later intervention. If one can act, for instance, on the mechanisms which lead to school maladjustment, one is in a stronger position to prevent the isolation, antisocial behaviour and possible delinquency of the children concerned and the adolescents they become. However, there is a paradox here and a danger, in that the earlier one acts in prevention, the more difficult it is to identify the children who will benefit most from the action. We shall elaborate on this in the second part of the chapter.

An interesting project in Mons (Belgium) is being undertaken by Pourtois and colleagues.[6] This project is based on the active intervention of the family in the process of educational help and, hence, of the successful readjustment to the learning activities. Another has been carried out in Maryland, the PICA project[7]—Programming Interpersonal Curricula for Adolescents—where in a school setting it proved possible to act on school failure and delinquent behaviour. In the longer term this programme proved successful in preventing social maladjustment.

One of the most interesting common denominators of several of these projects is that they rely to a large extent on self-help, help from neighbours, or on help from people in the same social community. The research psychologist or psychiatrist acts as a sort of catalyst and starts off a process which continues without any further professional input. However, while the effects of educational maladjustment and school failure are quite well known,[5] the long-term evaluation of preventive interventions are still to be carried out or, at least, to be completed.

Another interesting issue in this field is the prevention of psychosocial mental retardation, one of the main causes of school failure and of its later social consequences. Many interesting projects are currently in progress on this subject in various countries. The Head Start programme in the United States[8] has been very active in helping underprivileged families, mothers and children, to cope with educational issues, and to prevent the retardation process. Several groups have succeeded in improving performance, so that children previously attaining a development quotient (DQ) of about 80, have achieved levels of 100 or 120. This has been done at a very high cost, but the project apparently worked successfully. However the causes of these social inequalities have not yet been attacked, and the long-range results of such programmes are questionable.[9]

Social Health

The 'sociogenic' mental deficiency mentioned above is a concrete illustration of the huge question of social inequalities in the field of health, the ethical implications of which are quite obvious.

It is important to stress again the still heavy *inequalities* between populations—and children—of different social and economic groups, in the field of health and disease: death-rates, morbidity, occurrence of handicaps, of accidents, access to health services, and so on.

In France and in the United Kingdom the perinatal mortality ratio between the most and least privileged groups has not changed since the beginning of this century.[10] In Belgium, these differences have been confirmed recently.[11]

An urgent and difficult issue in the field of social medicine is how to reach the families and children of the most underprivileged social groups, the so-called 'Fourth World'.[12] There are important programmes underway in this field in several European countries including Belgium and France. Here again, the risk of using a normative approach is high. It is sometimes difficult indeed to understand the behaviour of people who see things so differently from ourselves and live in quite a different way. Values such as time, the keeping of appointments, the organization of life are often fundamentally different.

There is a very strong demand for freedom and dignity from and for this population. On this basis, important principles have been proposed in France by the Quart-Monde movement of Father Wresinski, which, almost as a prerequisite, points out the need for respect of the mental and social freedom of the underprivileged families and population.[13]

GENERAL PRINCIPLES AND PRACTICAL IMPLEMENTATION

It is first of all essential to recall the ethical rules governing all medical interventions—either curative or preventive—in paediatric practice, child care and medical research involving children.[14] However, these basic principles—'informed consent; potential usefulness; harmlessness; respect of cultural background; involvement of a doctor (mainly when research is involved); control mechanisms'—prepared for adults, are difficult to adapt to children who are usually considered in ethical codes along with insane and incapable people. In addition, chronological age, often used for defining the child's own level of responsibility, is a variable open to criticism. Use of the concept of mental age would be more accurate but it is difficult to have this taken into consideration in policy-making.

However, all ethical issues defined in preventive and social medicine for whole populations apply also to children. Moreover, principle 8 of the Declaration of the Rights of Children specifies: 'the child should, in all circumstances, be amongst the first ones to receive protection and care'. Let us consider, therefore, the advantages and disadvantages of this basic rule.

Children First?

The principle that the child should be among the first to receive protection and care has to be reassessed in the context of some very recent philosophical research in the United States on the legitimacy of the role of age in determining health care priorities—is age a legitimate criterion in deciding priorities?

Much thought has been stimulated by a sense that the very elderly get, or even deserve to get, low priority because of their age. Assuming that we are motivated by a commitment to provide equality of wellbeing among the population, it makes an enormous difference which of two possible interpretations is given.

According to the first one, we want equality of wellbeing at a given moment in time, in which case the infant and the elderly person would seem to get equal priority. An alternative interpretation is that we need equality of wellbeing over a lifetime. Since the elderly have had a great deal of care over much of their life, the direct implication of this argument is that the infant should get higher priority. This seems to apply directly to the above-mentioned principle and provides philosophical support for what may seem superficially to be a rather strange notion that the child deserves to be among the first to receive health protection and care.

One example of this approach is the effect of life expectancy upon our valuation of life—that is, the child is thought to be more valuable because it has longer to live. In this respect, the indiscriminate use of the indicator 'potential years of life lost' by any cause of death could be misleading. Paradoxically, when we move back to the fetus, say an 18 week fetus, this life expectancy effect seems to disappear. The fetus does not carry this valuation. That is a curiously illogical ambiguity or prejudice.

The Child in Crisis

Quite often, the child is a stake, and a victim, in conflicts between adults, between parents. Sometimes, his or her interests diverge from, and conflict with those of the parents. This can be the case in child abuse, including institutional abuse,[15] and in divorce. At national level in some countries, at worldwide level for those concerned with international child health, child victims of war, of sexual or work exploitation have to be protected by an enforced legislation and by necessary social changes.

The crisis situations threatening the health and sometime the life of the child plead for a child advocacy. This is the process by which children are protected by a competent adult from the adverse effects of these harmful conditions, and the role of the paediatrician as child advocate is certainly a crucial one.

What About Early Diagnosis?

Another basic principle has to do with the early diagnosis of potential handicapping conditions. It is assumed, in many instances, that the earlier the diagnosis, the easier the care and the better the result. This gives a background on which early medical or social interventions or both are based, since many disorders of adulthood or old age have their onset in childhood.[16] However, no such action should be undertaken without scientific evidence which is, in fact, very often lacking. As a consequence, guidelines and recommendations sometimes imposed on children and families become rapidly obsolescent, and are replaced by new ones that can be completely different. This has been humorously documented—as far as feeding rules and early education principles are concerned—in a French book entitled *L'art d'accommoder les bébés*.[17]

One can also argue that it is unethical to diagnose a condition if—according to current medical knowledge (or ignorance)—there is nothing to offer in order to alleviate the burden. Yet the lobbying of parents of handicapped children has, in many instances, stimulated the scientists as well as the policy-makers, and prompted progress towards better care.

Finally, by intervening early, we lose the ability to distinguish between those children who should be taken into preventive action and those who will cope efficiently with their problems by themselves. Let us recall the great variability of psychological conditions and troubles in childhood; many may be resolved without any professional intervention, and it might be unethical to 'medicalize', or to 'psychiatrize' these borderline mental health symptoms. In addition, too early an intervention makes it difficult to evaluate the effects of the treatment and care. There is no simple answer to this dilemma.[15]

The At Risk Strategy

Quite recently, a new strategy has been proposed to deal with health problems—be they physical, psychological or social in nature—the at risk approach which can be summed up very simply as 'health care for all, more for those more in need'.[18]

This strategy, however attractive, can sometimes be counterproductive, and lead to adverse effects, especially in the social field, where the 'labelling effect' and the victim blaming process constitute real dangers.

The underprivileged fringe of the population is frequently unable to protect itself from adverse measures (like the placement of children in institutions, foster homes) imposed upon it by society (the state), usually through social services. These measures are often detrimental, in terms of mental health, both for the children and for their parents. Consequently, the medical and social professions have to be aware of and to address the ethical issues raised by the following problems some of which are discussed in various contexts throughout this book: the rights of the individual versus the rights of society; the balance between rights and duties in all circumstances; the equilibrium to be found and kept between health protection (from outside) and health promotion (a personal commitment); the individuals and families 'left behind' by any health or social advance; the harmlessness of preventive measures—which can never be completely guaranteed; the reparation mechanisms that are to be developed to compensate for any injury resulting from the side-effects of preventive actions.[19] The latter point is also relevant to the somatic aspects of prevention, for example, immunization.

Screening—What For?

A common prejudice, which is perhaps more a medical than a society one, is that we tend to favour the prevention and treatment of discrete hazards with well-defined mechanisms. We understand the mechanisms of phenylketonuria, for example, and it has a discrete taxonomic diagnosis. Yet, there is a great deal we could do relatively simply in pregnancy and in the perinatal period to improve the intellectual and physical performance of our children. The use of effective education methods, for example, to reduce smoking in pregnancy and improve dietary intake, would increase birthweight and therefore reduce perinatal mortality and the risk of sensory and neuromotor defects. In numerical terms the benefit of this type of simple and inexpensive action far exceeds the benefit to be obtained from more costly investments in the prevention of phenylketonuria. Yet the one strategy is so highly valued that it would be unthinkable to withdraw screening for phenylketonuria and the other so undervalued that it is very difficult even to persuade an obstetrician to mention smoking or enquire about smoking habits.

In a study in France, reported by Senecal in 1982, for example, mass screening revealed 80 cases of phenylketonuria, but health statistics revealed 600 000 cases of maltreated or abandoned children, school absconders, drug addicts, suicide attempts and so on.[20] Similarly, in 1984, in Spain, a programme of mass screening identified 24 cases of phenylketonuria and over 35 000 cases of low birthweight.[20] Yet, medical training is focussed on the rare and virtually ignores the common facts of life to which doctors will be exposed in their daily practice. This imbalance must be a cause for concern and it raises again the question of priorities in decisions about large projects of prevention. The easiest to apply is not always the one that should be chosen.

Confidentiality and Dialogue

Confidentiality is increasingly and rightly emphasized, especially in the relationship between the doctor and the adolescent.[21] It may encompass confidentiality *vis-à-vis* the parents, sometimes a prerequisite for adolescents to trust their doctor. The age from which this confidential relationship should and could start is open to discussion, and certainly to variations.

On the same lines, one major problem in relation to the ethics of prevention in child health is that of communication of confidences between people of different disciplines, each relating professionally to a family where there is a child at risk. It may be the doctor, the community nurse, the social worker, the probation officer concerned with the family, the school doctor with an older child—each of these individuals may know of the possibility, for instance, of a child at risk of abuse, but feel bound by a strict interpretation of professional secrecy not to tell. This problem of secrecy between professional groups is a very difficult one, particularly in countries with a liberal medical tradition and a high regard for personal freedom. In some cities in Belgium—in Liège, for example, and Antwerp and Brussels—teams of health professionals have been set up to try to help in such situations. These are called 'équipes de confiance' and include doctors, nurses, and social workers, working together in a specified geographical area. Moreover, in France and in some other countries, doctors, nurses and social workers are not bound by professional secrecy when the life of a child is endangered by abusing adults.

This question of communication can be enlarged to include also the dialogue between medical and social research teams to try to improve health and social policy. The language of ethics as related to medicine is a language of normative and indicative statements. The language of politics is also normative, but prescriptive; there is at least some common ground between ethics and politics which could be further exploited to advantage. Regular channels of interdisciplinary communication could help to ensure that these political decisions will be based more firmly on the ethical and medical principles involved.

In cooperation between disciplines, sociology is a science which could be helpful in investigating ethical issues that arise from medical practice and research. Sociology, for example, can help in the diagnosis of socialization processes by which values about 'health and ill health' are transmitted in the family, at school, and through the mass media with obvious applications in health education. Here again, a common language has to be found.

Consent in Paediatric Practice and in Prevention

There is general agreement on the necessity of applying to paediatric practice as well as to preventive interventions the principles of 'informed consent'. However their effective implementation raises a number of serious problems, if only in defining the concept itself, as well as various practical constraints.[22–25]

First, it is difficult, if indeed possible at all, to define in clear terms the concept of informed consent.[26] Some authors, such as Jeanneret and Raymond, even use the word 'utopia'.[27] However, within the constraints that will be outlined here, definitions can be phrased only in general terms.[28]

At least two conditions are requested in the process of informed consent—a clear perception of the health problem at stake, whether curative or preventive, and the ability to decide in a responsible and autonomous way. For various reasons, in childhood as well as in adolescence, these conditions may not be fulfilled. One may wonder, incidentally, how often they are, even for adults! But what are the criteria of validity, considering on the one hand the child's or adolescent's abilities and on the other hand the health issue? The child should be able to perceive and to integrate the various dimensions and, often, the complexity of that issue.

Some authors feel that age level could be considered as a valid criterion. However, as far as specific age levels are suggested, they vary widely—for example, from 7 to 15.[25,28–31] Moreover, parents' reactions may prevent their children or even adolescents from expressing their opinions.[30]

Another suggestion concerns the IQ of the child which might be used, at least as a complementary source of information. But one should be aware of the relative validity of the appropriate testing techniques and it may be difficult to use tests when the informed consent of a child is requested.

The particular health problems involved raise other difficulties. Quite frequently the scientific knowledge required may be lacking or only partly available. How can we inform a child or a youngster about issues which are not clear to us[31,32] When data do exist, they may be difficult to explain in simple terms, without using epidemiological or statistical terminology, which may be clear for public health specialists and clinicians, but not intelligible to many people and, even less, to children. Nevertheless, these obstacles may be overcome if proper consideration is given to communication and to educational techniques used successfully, for example, in health education programmes. At any rate, an open discussion with the child, who should be free to ask questions, will be more efficient than a long monologue or a 'lecture' given by the physician.

Finally, the role of the parents and of their own consent must be considered carefully. In the case of very young children, parental consent has to be obtained.[31] Even with mature children and adolescents, it may be helpful in the majority of cases that the parents give their advice and their consent as well.

Difficulties may develop whenever there is a disagreement or even a conflict between the parents and their child.[33] In some cases medical treatment may be accepted by the latter but not by the parents.[34] Medical care may be requested by an adolescent, for example, in the field of mental health without the consent of the parents,[35] who may even ignore the situation altogether as is often the case in family planning clinics. In some cases one may evoke the intervention of a 'child advocate' as has happened dramatically in the instance of battered children.[36]

These are some of the more frequently observed situations which do not contradict the general necessity of respecting the child's freedom and autonomy to consent, whenever possible. But there is no magic formula suggesting answers to the great variety and the complexity of the issues to be considered. We may conclude, with Raimbault, that the attitude of the parents and the health personnel may enable the child to work out his personal 'research'.[30] 'One of the major ethical problems in paediatrics concerns precisely the attitude to this "research" (questionnement), which means the child's appeal to its very existence'.

RESEARCH AND TRAINING

Is Paediatric Research Ethical?

It is sometimes argued that research should not be carried out in children, even in areas where the risk would be relatively minimal, precisely because the children cannot give informed consent. The extension of this argument is surely that increasingly effective, non-dangerous medicine is only for consenting adults.

Research is of course essential for progress in the field of child health as in any other. And such research is questioned on moral rather than medical grounds. The ethical dilemma here involves the risk attached to its application to children.

In assessing the viability of a given research project, the risk is measured against the benefit. In this context there is an important distinction between therapeutic and non-therapeutic research. The former is for the benefit of the patient or subject himself, the latter may provide more benefit for others.

In this difficult context, one has indeed to keep to a minimum the amount of research in children and to allow nothing beyond minimal risk. The National Commission for the Protection of Human Subjects of Biomedical and Behavioural Research in the United States defines minimal risk as that which is normally encountered in daily living or in the routine medical or psychological examination of healthy children. Even so defined, minimal is a relative term, and the Committees of Ethics dealing with research problems should be especially cautious when research projects—in the medical as well as in the social field—involve children.

Teaching Ethics?

There is a need to sensitize future physicians and health professionals to social and ethical issues involved in the practice of medicine and to include appropriate topics, such as social sciences, philosophy, ethics, in their curriculum as is already done in some countries.[14]

There is also a need for continuous education in this field, especially for those professionals facing some difficult ethical situation in their current work, or being constantly confronted with quite different value systems which make their work complicated. Some of these issues are impossible to solve without specific training and much thought and discussion.

Finally, one must also consider the ethics of teaching and training medical students and where the emphasis should lie in order to prevent some of what we can call the new morbidity or new pathology in developed countries.

REFERENCES

1. Manciaux, M. Ethique et vaccination des enfants. *Sciences sociales et Santé* 1984; **2**: 168–189.
2. Manciaux, M. and Tomkiewicz, S. *Mental deficiency in the young*. Paris: INSERM, 1983.
3. Sand, E. A. Agressivité. **In**: *Les adolescents et leur santé*. Paris: Flammarion Médecine-Sciences, 1983: 226–237.
4. Soumenkoff, G., Marneffe, C., Gerard, M. *et al.* A coordinated attempt for prevention of child abuse at the antenatal care level. *Child Abuse and Neglect* 1982; **6**: 87–94.

5. Sand, E. A., Hauzeur, C., Roger, G. *et al. L'echec scolaire à l'école primaire. Aspects psychosociaux—Prévention*. Bruxelles: Ministère de l'Education nationale et de la Culture française. Direction Générale de l'Organisation des Etudes, Collection Recherche en Education, 1982, **21**: 134; **22**: 121.
6. Pourtois, J. P. *et al. Recherches sur les handicaps socio-culturels de 0 à 7–8 ans*. Bruxelles: Ministère de l'Education nationale et de la Culture française. Direction Générale de l'Organisation des Etudes, Collection Recherche en Education, 1973, **1**: 450.
7. PICA Project. *Programming Interpersonal Curricula for Adolescents*. Washington DC: National Institute of Mental Health, Center for Studies of Crime and Delinquency, 1970.
8. *Head Start in the 1980s*. A report requested by the President of the United States. HMS, 1980, 393.
9. Manciaux, M. and Tomkiewicz, S. *Facteurs socio-économiques et culturels associés aux différentes formes de la déficience mentale chez l'enfant*. Quebec: Presses de l'Université du Québec (in press).
10. Manciaux, M., Rumeau-Rouquette, C. Morbidité et mortalité périnatale: Approche épidémiologique. **In**: Vert, P. Stern, L. (eds). *Médecine Néonatale*. Paris: Masson, 1985: 3–44.
11. Lagasse, R. *Les déterminants de la morbidité maternelle et infantile*. Thèse d'agrégation de l'enseignement supérieur. Bruxelles: Université Libre de Bruxelles, Faculté de Médecine, 1985.
12. Houtaud, (d') A. *La santé des enfants et des familles du Quart-monde dans les pays industrialisés (approche bibliographique)*. Paris: Centre International de l'Enfance, 1983.
13. ATD Quart-Monde. *Vivre dans la dignité*. Méry sur Oise: Sciences et Services, 1985.
14. Royer, P. and Guignard, J. *Ethique et Pédiatrie*. Paris: Flammarion Médecine-Sciences, 1981.
15. Straus, P., Manciaux, M. and Deschamps, G. *L'Enfant Maltraité*. Paris: Fleurus, 1982.
16. Falkner, F. *Prevention in Childhood of Health Problems in Adult Life*. Geneva: World Health Organisation 1980.
17. Delaisy de Parseval, G. and Lallemand, N. *L'Art d'Accommoder les Bébés*. Paris: Seuil, 1980.
18. Backett, E. M., Davies, A. M. and Petros-Barvazian, A. *Risk approach in health care, with special reference to maternal and child health*. Geneva: World Health Organisation. Public Health Papers, 1984, **76**.
19. Ratcliffe, J., Wallack, L., Fagnani, F. *et al*. Perspectives on Prevention: Health Promotion as Health Protection. **In**: de Kervasdoué, J., Kimberley, J. R., Rodwin, V. G. (eds). *The End of an Illusion*. Berkeley: University of California Press, 1984: 35–54.
20. Senecal, J. Personal Communication, 1985.
21. Jeanneret, O., Sand, E. A., Deschamps, J. P. *et al. Les Adolescents et Leur Santé*. Paris: Flammarion Médecine-Sciences, 1983.
22. Jeanneret, O. and Raymond, L. Ethique médicale et épidémiologie expérimentale. Considérations sur les études d'intervention chez l'enfant et l'adolescent. *Rev Epidémiol Santé Publique* 1978; **26**: 479–499.
23. Melton, G., Koocher, G., Saks, M. (eds.) *Children's Competence to Consent*. Plenum Press, 1983.
24. Royer, P. Ethique des essais thérapeutiques et des recherches scientifiques poursuivis chez les mineurs. *Arch Fr Pédiatr* 1979; **36**: 333–338.
25. Working party on ethics of research in children: guidelines to aid ethical committees considering research involving children. *Br Med J* 1980; **280**: 229–231.

26. Kumate, J. Etica de la investigacion en pediatria. **In**: *Medical Ethics and Medical Education*. Vol 1, Geneva: Council for International Organizations of Medical Sciences. 1981: 129–136.
27. Jeanneret, O. and Raymond, L. Aspects éthiques des études d'intervention. *Rev Epidémiol et Santé Publique* 1981; **29**: 269–279.
28. Jonsen, A. R. Research involving children: Recommendations of the National Commission for the Protection of Human Subjects of Biomedical and Behavioral Research. *Pediatrics* 1978; **62**: 131–136.
29. Committee on Drugs. Guidelines for the ethical conduct of studies to evaluate drugs in pediatric population. *Pediatrics* 1977; **60**: 91–101.
30. Raimbault, G. Le soutien psychologique à l'enfant chroniquement malade et à sa famille: aspects éthiques. **In**: Royer P, Guignard, J. (eds). *Ethique et Pédiatrie*. Paris: Flammarion Médecine Sciences, 1982.
31. Skegg, P. D. G. English law relating to experimentation on children. *Lancet* 1977; **2**: 754–755.
32. Eisenberg, L. The social imperatives of medical research. *Science* 1977; **198**: 1105-1110.
33. Committee on Youth. The implications of minor's consent legislation for adolescent health care: a commentary. *Pediatrics* 1974; **54**: 481–485.
34. Shaw, A. Dilemmas of 'Informed Consent' in children. *N Engl J Med* 1973; **289**: 885-890.
35. Schowalter, J. E. The minor's role in consent for mental health treatment. *J Child Psychiatr* 1978; **17**: 505–513.
36. Serota, F. T., August, C. S. Tuohy O'Shea, A. *et al*. Role of a child advocate in the selection of donors for pediatric bone marrow transplantation. *J Pediatr* 1981; **98**: 847–850.

Ethical Dilemmas in Health Promotion
Edited by S. Doxiadis

CHAPTER 14

Mass Screening Procedures and Programmes

POVL RIIS

SUMMARY

Ethical aspects of mass screening can be analysed from two angles—that of the citizen as an individual and that of society as a whole. The individual has to face a potential conflict between his autonomy and safety on the one hand and the benefits he may gain from innovations in mass screening on the other. Society's aim in this context is the protection of the state and its citizens and the promotion of health. In planning health promotion a central ethical question arises—how far can society go in accepting the self-destruction of certain citizens by damaging habits and life-styles, some of which may even impose a risk on other people? The chapter presents a framework for ethical analyses of mass screening programmes. Seven key questions need to be answered: (1) Is the programme part of a scientific project? (2) Can the individual citizen expect a personal benefit? (3) Has informed consent been obtained? (4) Is the programme national or international? (5) Which subgrouping of health stages are involved? (6) Which subgrouping of life periods are involved? (7) Will the programme inflict secondary ethical dilemmas of resource allocation? Examples of analyses are taken from antenatal diagnostic procedures, genetic screening in high risk families, and screening for viral hepatitis antigens and antibodies. The chapter concludes with the suggested creation in each country of a Central Advisory Ethical Committee, attached to the Ministry of Health or the Interior, comprising an equal number of lay and so-called professional members. Today not only a dialogue, but continuous cooperation of such a direct kind is seriously needed, to secure the proper exploitation of scientific guidance and the representation of ethical concern in future mass screening and other preventive measures.

DEFINITIONS

I will begin by defining the key concepts of my title—'Mass screening procedures and programmes—ethical issues'.

In the context of this book mass *screening* is defined as *large scale diagnosis*. Thus, the diagnostic procedure involved in screening does not start from the usual patient–doctor contact. On the contrary, individually screened persons' contact with the health system is determined from outside, on a non-individual level. *Mass* as a quantitative character means *involving substantial fractions of, or whole, population groups*, representative according to sex, age, profession and so on.

By *procedures* I mean *the diagnostic methods in a practical sense*, as applied to individual citizens, and a *programme* is defined as *an administrative campaign*, planned and implemented by central health authorities.

Ethical describes *the sum of fundamental principles underlying human value judgments* (with *morals* being the practical implementation in daily life of such principles).

Issues or *aspects* in this context cover *the possible ethical problems of the public interventions in question*, as seen through the process of ethical analysis.

PRINCIPAL ETHICAL ASPECTS

Mass screening procedures and programmes will have to be analysed from two different angles, that of the individual citizen and that of the society.

The *individual* in European countries (and probably even in a global context) will stress his or her right to (1) self-determination or autonomy, (2) security or safety, and (3) the benefits of medical progress in terms of diagnosis, treatment and prevention. *Society* will emphasize its responsibility for preventing or counteracting health catastrophes, for instance large epidemics, and for intervening in order to increase the health standard of its citizens. In the following these ethical demands will be discussed separately.

Individual rights to *self-determination* or autonomy have been strongly reinforced by the citizens' rights movement which started in the late 1960s and has continued until now. The compatibility of self-determination with the fundamental democratic principles of European constitutions is obvious, but the citizens' rights movement has without doubt contributed substantially to the implementation of such rights in society. The movement strongly influenced matters such as education, working conditions and health, and, as a part of the health sector, biomedical research and preventive programmes.

Besides self-determination, people have a right to *security* or *safety*. This implies that involvement in interventions planned and executed by those in authority will have to be safe—that is, people must not be exposed to any risk. But safety also involves protection from undue risks caused by neighbours or fellow citizens, especially in terms of serious contagious diseases. In this way the ethical interests of citizen and society run parallel instead of being antagonistic.

Autonomy and safety are protected by the technique of *informed consent*. By initially informing the individual of a planned programme and asking him or her to participate, citizens will know if mass programmes—or any other medical intervention—take place, and at what cost.

The third ethical principle applied by individuals is the right to benefit from innovations in mass screening and a resulting intervention, if necessary. But this understandable expectation brings about a conflict of interests. On the one hand the wish for autonomy and safety in the short term might prevent the progress of clinical science. On the other hand, progress of medical science in the long term presupposes cooperation with the citizens, even to the extent of reducing the demand for maximum safety (after informed consent of course). Such opposing motives can reach a schizophrenic stage, but this happens rarely because few people are willing or sufficiently knowledgeable to face both perspectives.

Societies' ethical attitudes deal with *protection* and *health promoting regulation*.

Protection from mass health disasters can lead to interventions involving temporary reduction of individual citizens' rights—for instance isolation, obligatory examinations or vaccinations. Such rare interventions will be justified by the principle of *jus necessitatis* that is, the state acts in order to secure its, and its citizens', survival.

Less dramatic, and more common, are the means applied to preserve or increase—that is *regulate*—the health status of society. The mass programme of the World Health Organization, *Health for All by the Year 2000*,[4] reflects this ethical aspect in several ways. In this context one can ask how far society can go in accepting self-destruction of some individuals by damaging habits and life-styles, even to the extent of imposing a risk on others?

ETHICAL GUIDELINES

Which rules determine the ethical acceptability of mass screening programmes? At present no international sets of guidelines (and probably not even national ones) exist to regulate this important field.

The Second Helsinki Declaration of 1975[2] and the Proposed International Guidelines for Biomedical Research Involving Human Subjects[3] of the Council for International Organizations of Medical Sciences (CIOMS) are both guidelines for *scientific* ethics. Yet the fundamental ethical attitudes involved in the Declaration and the Guidelines will be valid even for the non-experimental areas of mass screening programmes.

The Second Helsinki Declaration does not explicitly mention preventive measures, but such interventions are considered to be covered by their elements of diagnosis or treatment. The Declaration stresses the importance of risk assessments and informed consent. The Declaration also states that 'concern for the interests of the subject must always prevail over the interest of science and society'.

On the item 'community-based research', The Council for International Organizations of Medical Sciences deals mainly with *therapeutic* intervention, again from the *scientific* point of view, but this is still very relevant even for non-experimental programmes:[1,3]

> 'The provision of basic prophylactic care on a community basis is the aim and the obligation of every public health service. These measures, moreover, are often accorded force of law on the thesis that any incidental infringement of individual liberties is decisively outweighed by benefit to the community as a whole. In some instances this care commits individuals, either singly or collectively, to exposure to biologically active substances. Compulsory vaccination and implementation of vector control programmes offer obvious examples while addition of iodide to table salt, of vitamins to staple foods, of nitrate to meat products and of fluoride to public water supplies further illustrates the scope of such provisions. The benefits are incontestable, but apprehension concerning risks—both hypothetical and apparent—has, on occasion, obstructed their acceptance.'

Here the guidelines accept a kind of State paternalism, allowing the state to infringe on individual liberties if the benefits to society seem to outweigh such infringements. The most important perspective is the acceptance of such an outcome under certain circumstances. The inborn weakness is of course the difficulty in defining a balance point between 'benefit' and necessary 'infringement'.

The guidelines state further:

> 'Wherever interventionist public health policies are accepted as a function of government, a complementary need to assess and to monitor the consequences of such measures from the time they are planned—and for as long as they remain in operation—must be accepted not only by the responsible authorities, but by the community at large. Observations on considerable numbers of subjects are usually required if reliable estimates of performance, both beneficial and adverse, are to be obtained. Moreover, these effects may be measurable only in terms of a collective response and comparisons between treated and untreated communities may be required to discern them'.

The obligation of linking intervention programmes—whether planned as research projects or not—to follow-up monitoring is clearly stressed. The reasons seem obvious, to evaluate the outcome with the larger perspective of exploiting the results for the benefit of other such groups, and to analyse the ethical consequences of State paternalism. The need for doing such assessments with research methods is emphasized not surprisingly in a set of *scientific*-ethical guidelines.

Special problems are related to comparative field projects in developing countries, especially when authorities or scientists from developed countries are involved: 'These considerations apply with even greater force in many developing countries where comparative field trials undertaken on a community basis frequently offer the only practicable means of objectively determining policies relating to issues as diverse as nutritional requirements, environmental and/or occupational health regulations, vaccination programmes and other measures applied in the control of communicable disease.'

The Guidelines openly deal with the problem of obtaining informed consent in field projects:

> 'When it is impracticable to elicit adequately-informed consent from every individual implicated in a field study, investigations, can only proceed upon the basis of meticulous assessment, competent technical advice, and an acceptable procedure for delegation of the power of consent from the individual subject to an independent representative body charged to protect community interests. The precise mechanisms through which delegation of consent is achieved will be influenced by political philosophy, the nature and inter-relationships of governmental and professional institutions, the degree of centralization of administrative processes, the structure of society, cultural precepts, and the degree of sophistication of the communities directly involved in the matters at issue. The responsibility for such community-based studies must rest, directly or indirectly, with government agencies.'

The serious ethical problem of consent delegation has an obvious parallel in clinical research on minors, the mentally retarded, and so on.

Another parallel with clinical research is the importance of not involving more subjects in a given intervention project than is necessary for obtaining a valid result. This principle is applicable even in non-experimental intervention campaigns, if any doubt on their effectiveness remains: 'Having regard to the inherent difficulties, community-based research should be entertained only when the expectation of benefit to the community is adequately secure and when smaller-scale studies would not produce a conclusive result'.

After these statements in the general survey, the Guidelines themselves state the following:

> '16 Where research is undertaken on a community basis—for example by experimental treatment of water supplies, by health services research or by large-scale trials of new insecticides, of new prophylactic or immunizing agents, and of nutritional adjuvants or substitutes—individual consent on a person-to-person basis may not be feasible, and the ultimate decision to undertake the research will rest with the responsible public health authority.
>
> 17 Nevertheless, all possible means should be used to inform the community concerned of the aims of the research, the advantages expected from it, and any possible hazards or inconveniences. If feasible, dissenting individuals should have the option of withholding their participation. Whatever the circumstances,

the ethical considerations and safeguards applied to research on individuals must be translated, in every possible respect, into the community context'.

STRUCTURED ETHICAL ANALYSES OF MASS SCREENING PROGRAMMES

As with research ethics and clinical ethics, there is a need for a structured analysis technique when mass screening programmes are to be evaluated ethically.[4,5,6,7] There are seven key questions which require to be answered and I will now consider these in turn.

1 Is the Programme Part of a Scientific Project or Not?

There is a strong need for screening programmes to be tested scientifically. Yet such programmes are still started without a built-in possibility for valid scientific evaluation of its costs and benefits. Thus, both types of mass screening take place to-day.

If the mass screening involves a contemporary control group allowing the responsible authorities to evaluate the programme, then the Second Helsinki Declaration and the CIOMS Proposed International Guidelines have advised on the ethical standards. Accordingly the public will have to be informed, and the individual citizen asked to participate, with an undebatable right to refuse to take part.

If the mass screening is non-experimental (even if it ought to be) the citizens' right to abstain ought to be the same as in the case of scientific projects. However, not all countries express such a right explicitly, and sometimes there is indirect pressure for participation—'it is a programme for everyone', 'it is a valuable offer, so why not enter it?'.

2 Can the Individual Citizen Expect a Personal Benefit?

This question will have to be answered in terms of a health benefit, and not in terms as fulfilling 'the duties of a good citizen'. The benefit will have to be evaluated as the difference between benefits *and risks*.

If the answer to this question is no, the ethical implications will be much more severe, because the citizen's risk will have to be balanced against society's gain, a comparison difficult to make because no overall unity for such measurements exists. The citizen's risk/society's benefit discussion will have to be taken in the open, involving the media and the general public.

3 Has Informed Consent Been Obtained?

As already discussed in question 1, informed consent is a basic demand, whether the programme is experimental or not. But the question has to be put explicitly, as a part of a check-list applied when mass screening programmes are ethically evaluated.

As is the case in certain active intervention programmes—for instance, water fluoridation programmes—informed consent, as in the usual patient-doctor relationship, is not possible. Even in diagnostic programmes, for example, mass screening for certain antibody titres in the population, if common blood samples collected clinically for a completely different purpose, are analysed in a central national laboratory, the test subjects will not have consented. They might even find out about the programme by being approached secondarily because of their personal test results.

Like informed consent in the case of scientific projects in community medicine, consent is sometimes not accessible in countries with a subtle infrastructure or a substantial degree of illiteracy or both. Informed consent in mass programmes in developed countries will sometimes have to be given indirectly—that is by proxy. How this can be organized will be discussed in a later section of this chapter.

4 Is the Programme National or International?

The answer to this question will often be national, which means that the programme takes place in one's own country. If, however, the programme is organized by the home country but takes place in another country, for instance a developing country, other ethical aspects arise. Not only is it necessary that the receiving country analyses and accepts the programme on behalf of its citizens, but also the sending—or organizing—country will have to deal with the ethical implications. As a rule both countries' authorities will have to be responsible for the programme's ethical standards. Once more the operational approach to this problem will be touched upon later in this chapter.

5 Which Subgrouping of Health Stages are Involved?

Does the screening comprise so-called *risk groups* (for instance members of certain families or professions), *pre-illness groups or early morbid cases*, the last two found in the general population? The ethics involved in the screening programmes will vary accordingly. The strongest motivation will be met in the risk groups, but at the same time the ethical dilemma for the individual group member will vary widely with the existence or the non-existence of a treatment or effective prevention.

The mere existence of a screening programme in small identifiable risk groups, will sometimes stigmatize the group's members, whether they participate in the screening or not, and whether the result of an individual screening test is disclosed or not. If stigmatization can be avoided and the anonymity of data preserved, screening data can be exploited for epidemiological purposes.

6 Which Subgrouping of Life Periods are Involved?

Life periods can be *prenatal*, *antenatal* or *postnatal*, the latter being further subdivided between children and adults (with further subgrouping being possible—for instance the elderly).

Antenatal screening can in rare cases lead to treatment of the unborn child, or more often to immediate intervention after birth. But in most cases a severe antenatal diagnosis will lead to legal abortion. Needless to say, such an intervention is fortunately unknown in postnatal cases. Thus, the differences in ethical concern vary to a large extent between the two main groups. The ethical aspects of antenatal screening will be discussed later.

7 Will the Programme Inflict Secondary Ethical Dilemmas of Resource Allocation?

Even in the most affluent societies, the health budget has an upper limit. This means that new demands, derived from scientific innovations or from needs unmasked through screening, will create pressure on already existing budget entries. If such a pressure is resisted politically the results of the screening can not be transformed into intervention. In such a situation the citizens are left with a feeling of frustration through having obtained information relevant to their health without the possibility of exploiting it. An example of such ethical aspects of health economy allocations will be given.

EXAMPLES OF ETHICAL ANALYSES

Antenatal Diagnosis in High Risk Families Versus Mass Antenatal Screening

Screening offered to risk families[6] raises fewer ethical problems than mass screening.[8] Risk families can be outlined by the mother's or the father's high age (related to the appearance of Down's Syndrome), the birth of previous children with severe, inherited defects and so on. Grave ethical problems can be involved here, when the test result is to be used in practical decision-making. Can the information be presented in a truly objective way? Do small defects have to be reported, if they are found by chance and how small is small? Is the sex of the unborn child to be disclosed if sex is of no importance for detecting a given disease or defect? What happens if the mother refuses an offer of abortion? Will society change its attitude towards congenital defects, from fate to avoidable conditions in the future?

Mass antenatal screening will further increase the ethical problems, especially on where to set the thresholds for defects or morbid genes. There is the possibility that such programmes will encourage expectations of perfection in childbearing as a human right similar to the degree of perfection expected when buying a new car.

At worst we might even fear that society's attitude towards congenital defects will change, especially in cases where families have not accepted the offer of antenatal screening, or, have turned down a resulting offer of legal abortion. Supportive measures from society to a family having a child with a congenital defect are often expensive, making the influence of an unexploited prevention critical.

Genetic Screening in Risk Families

Such screening can be applied as part of a scientific project or can represent a practical application of a proven method. It can further exemplify screening for ongoing disease (for instance, familial hyperlipidemia) or for genetic markers indicating the later appearance of a disease (for instance, Huntington's chorea). To emphasize the complexity of such ethical analyses, genetic screening in risk families can be antenatal, as in example 1, with induced abortion as the major intervention, or postnatal with quite different consequences in terms of prognostic insight.

In the years to come, postnatal genetic screening is expected to be available on a large scale, primarily because of increasing numbers of DNA-probes for precise genetic mapping of risk regions.

Huntington's chorea represents a characteristic example. The underlying genetic defect has not been located. Instead nearby base sequences seem to create promising possibilities for diagnosing the later appearance of Huntington's chorea in a given person.

Screening with the scientific purpose of testing the genetic markers involves research ethics in accordance with the Second Helsinki Declaration. If the detection of markers is shown to be reliable, screening as a practical implementation, offered to all Huntington families will raise very serious ethical problems. The mere existence of such screening methods will change the younger family members' and their parents' and partners' attitude. Would it be worthwhile to open the 'dark box' and find the truth—cruel as it would be in 50 per cent of cases, or relieving in the rest? Would the unmovable truth of carrying Huntington's chorea not be detrimental to the life of the individual before the age of 40–45 years when the disease usually starts? Or would the opposite be true in some patients? Would the knowledge of being a carrier positively influence the attitude towards childbearing, involving donor insemination in male cases and egg donation in female cases? Can one risk the possibility that authorities or employers might demand genetic screening in Huntington family members before they could be appointed? Are we ready to manage the situation that certain facts of a person's future, once given, can never be neutralized? The perspectives of genetic mass screening are certainly formidable.

Screening For Viral Hepatitis Antigens and Antibodies

This example highlights yet another ethical dimension of mass screening programmes, in the present case a future programme. Viral hepatitis of type B is one of the real health scourges of today. This disease causes not only a huge amount of acute illness but is also responsible for chronic liver disease and there is a strong suspicion that hepatitis B virus is the underlying cause of liver cancer in the developing countries.

Screening for the presence of HB_sAg and anti-HB_s would be valuable as mass screening *if* those being negative for both could be offered vaccination against hepatitis B. Such mass vaccination *after* screening would have a great preventive effect, not only measured in prevented acute hepatitis cases, but also probably as a large-scale cancer preventive intervention.

But, the ethical dimension here is of a economic nature. The cost of one series of vaccine injections is at present approximately US $ 120–140, and given the number of HB_sAg/Anti-HB_s-negative people, the cost of application of a mass vaccine programme would be prohibitive, even in the affluent Western societies. Consequently, until very cheap vaccines are reproduced by a recombinant DNA technique or an amino-acid sequence synthesis, it will be impossible to convert the detection of HB_sAg/Anti-HB-negativity by screening to an efficient vaccine prophylaxis. Screening without such a natural consequence will normally lead to frustration and is ethically questionable. Economic scarcity, whether relative or absolute, in this way lies behind the ethical conflict.

ETHICAL CONTROL OF MASS SCREENING PROGRAMMES—PRACTICAL ASPECTS

Not many years have passed since health authorities and the health professions arranged mass screenings (or other interventions) relying only on the organizers' own ethical judgment—if such a judgment and the underlying ethical analysis were even made conscious. The organizers of those days were not in any way acting deliberately unethically within the current framework of paternalism. One can only note that today's psychological climate between health authorities and the health professions demands much more information and much more self-determination before large-scale screening programmes can be launched.

What would be an appropriate way of organizing such ethical analyses in practice? Normally, Ministries of Health have the final responsibility for mass screening programmes. Consequently it might seem natural to place the necessary ethical evaluations of community medical interventions within these ministries or related agencies. Such a classical solution will, however, carry with it certain drawbacks. The most important of these will be the closed management of ethical questions since openness is considered to be central in the dialogue between health authorities and public opinion. If only for this reason, such a centralized administrative system will probably be considered unacceptable.

This leads us to consider other principles and models. One such model would be to refer all mass screening programmes, being part of a scientific project, to a competent scientific-ethical committee—and for those countries which have a central, national committee with strong lay representation this body could serve as a natural basis for this. Further, it would be possible to refer non-project linked screening programmes to a new body, called for instance the Central Advisory Ethical Committee, attached to the Ministry of Health or the Ministry of the Interior with a certain inbuilt autonomy. Such a new body would have to include as members medically competent people and an equal number of lay people (or equal plus one).

Ethical questions related to mass screening could be presented to the Committee either by Ministries or by other authorities (or even Parliament). Equally the Committee itself could take the initiative to start a public discussion and make its own statements and recommendations which would of course *not* be binding on either the parliament or the ministries or agencies involved.

The risk involved in such a construction would be that the Committee might become involved in minor political quarrels on resource distribution described as 'ethical problems' in order to lift them to a sphere of solemnity and importance. If that were to happen the Committee would not be able to serve its original purpose, to be the citizens' guarantee for the necessary inclusion of ethical premisses in the planning of major health interventions.

Not only a dialogue but also continuous cooperation of a more direct kind is seriously needed in this particular area of preventive medicine, now and in the future. The good old days of administrative paternalism have disappeared for good—a fact to be welcomed by politicians, administrators and doctors who must now cooperate to create and exploit scientific guidance for mass screening and other preventive measures.

REFERENCES

1. Council for International Organizations of Medical Sciences. Bankowski, Z. and Howard-Jones, N. (eds). *Human Experimentation and Medical Ethics*. Geneva: CIOMS, 1982.

2. World Medical Association. *The Helsinki Declaration II* (1975 version). Tokyo: WMA, 1985.
3. Council for International Organizations of Medical Sciences. *Proposed International Guidelines for Biomedical Research Involving Human Subjects*. Geneva: CIOMS, 1982.
4. World Health Organization: *Health for All by the Year 2000*. Geneva: WHO, 1984.
5. Martin, J. F. Potential and limits of health legislation, with particular respect to prevention. Eimeren, W. V., Engelbrecht, R. and Flagle, C. D. (eds). **In**: *Third Conference on System Science in Health Care*. Berlin-Heidelberg: Springer, 1984.
6. The Ministry of the Interior, Denmark (In Danish). *Fremskridtets pris: etiske problemer ved gensplejsning, aeg-transplantation, kunstig befrugtning og fosterdiagnostik*. Copenhagen: Indenrigsministeriet, 1984.
7. President's Commission for the study of Ethical Problems in Medical and Biomedical and Behavioural Research. *Summing Up: the Ethical and Legal Problems in Medicine and Biomedical and Behavioural Research*. Washington: PCSEPMBBR, 1983.
8. Riis, P. and Fuchs, F. Antenatal determination of foetal sex in prevention of hereditary diseases. *Lancet* 1960; **2**: 180–2.

Ethical Dilemmas in Health Promotion
Edited by S. Doxiadis

CHAPTER 15

Ethical Aspects of Prevention Trials

T. STRASSER, O. JEANNERET, AND L. RAYMOND

SUMMARY

Policy decisions in preventive medicine should be based on the results of prevention trials. Investigators involved in such trials carry a high social and ethical responsibility. This responsibility needs to be clearly defined and judiciously distributed among the protagonists of a trial, while the identity and unity of the responsible scientific body should be preserved. As in medical ethics in general, the theoretical bases and guiding principles in prevention trials are, respect for other people, beneficence, justice, informed consent, information, and systematic assessment of risks and benefits. There are, however, a number of special considerations, such as the complexity of ethical aspects of prevention studies, informed consent of whole populations or groups, age-related questions, the responsibility of interpreting the results of prevention studies, and potential clashes with some socio-cultural values. The underlying, central ethical issues—pertinent to the whole field of preventive medicine—are the disparity between individual autonomy and public interest, society's values of health and, in particular, the medical profession's commitment to prevention. The latter is considered a deontological imperative.

INTRODUCTION

Prevention trials are controlled studies designed and carried out with the purpose of obtaining objective information on the effects of preventive measures; they are intended to constitute the scientific basis of public health policies and decisions in preventive medicine. The preventive measures evaluated by such studies include a wide array of interventions, such as environmental engineering or protection, food and water additives, vaccination, mass screening, the use of drugs for the purpose of primary or secondary prevention, behavioural (life-style) modifications, and health education. *Intervention trials* have been defined by McMahon[1] as 'a cohort study in which the difference between cohorts is in respect to some artificially introduced characteristics'; the term in its generic sense therefore largely overlaps with 'prevention trials', but is in current usage rather restricted to behavioural interventions. In this chapter we deal with studies of preventive measures (interventions) in the broadest sense of the term. However, the examples to be discussed will be taken mostly from cardiovascular prevention, since it is a topical and expanding, if controversial, field.

The differences and similarities between clinical (therapeutic) and epidemiological (preventive) trials have been discussed elsewhere.[2-4] There are many published reports on the ethical difficulties of clinical trials (for example,[5-11]) with a feeling of a crisis,[12] even an impasse, occasionally emerging.[13] On the other hand, publications on ethical problems in preventive trials are scarce[4] and methodological considerations of such studies, covering ethical aspects[14] are exceptional.

DIFFERENCES BETWEEN ETHICAL CONSIDERATIONS IN CLINICAL AND PREVENTION TRIALS

It may be useful to recapitulate the differences between clinical (therapeutic) and preventive action. The clinical situation is based on the individual doctor-patient relationship; it is a concrete, relatively easily definable, direct interaction in which the physician carries an immediate responsibility for his decisions and acts, facing the patient directly (the parents in the case of a child, the family if the patient's consciousness is impaired); only secondarily is the doctor more or less responsible to society as intermediary of this personal act.

On the other hand, as a public health issue, prevention usually implies mass action, often the exposure of whole populations to measures to be decided upon by a body of medical or, more typically, non-medical decision-makers, advised by health scientists. The responsibility of taking or, for that matter, of not taking a decision radically differs from that in the clinical situation. Individual responsibility may be diluted or covered up by the fact that the decision is usually a collective one. In some situations moreover the interest of the individual may be at variance with that of society. The terms of the 'contract' between patient and physician are no longer valid in such collective preventive actions, although one could envisage a 'collective contract' between society and the health professions; this would then imply also a collective responsibility, a rather doubtful category. It may be that the fact that responsibility has often become collective is one of the sources of the perceived 'dehumanization' of clinical medicine.

The ethical inferences of all this for prevention trials are of prime importance. Prevention trials are, almost by definition, of high social relevance, and thus of considerable ethical importance, by virtue of the sheer numbers of people potentially influenced by the outcome of the study. And to this should be added the ethical value of disease prevention itself, with interest in larger rather than smaller numbers of patients. Since prevention trials are usually cooperative undertakings carried out by large teams, it is important ethically that neither the responsibility for nor the merit of such a study should be allowed to disappear by fragmentation but that it should be distributed judiciously among the participants, while preserving the unity and identity of the responsible body.

SELECTED ETHICAL ISSUES IN PREVENTION TRIALS

In this chapter we cannot attempt to cover all ethical problems arising in intervention trials. The theoretical bases and guiding principles are those of medical ethics in general, as described in the Belmont Report:[15] respect for persons, beneficence, justice, as well as informed consent, information, and systematic assessment of risks and benefits. The latter is best done by building into the study protocol a statistical method called 'sequential analysis', which allows continuous monitoring of both positive and negative effects, and calls for terminating the study as soon as preset statistical significance has been achieved either on the positive or on the negative side. This has become a standard method ever since its introduction by Armitage several decades ago. It is obvious (though it may not always be realized) that good scientific methodology is an essential also of the ethics of any study. Only a trial with a sound scientific basis can be an ethical trial—although, of course, good science *per se* is not a guarantee of good ethics.

With regard to prevention studies, however, some special considerations need emphasis. Prevention studies may raise particularly complex ethical issues. Informed consent calls for additional reflection in prevention studies. The age of the study cohort members, whether very young or very old, may pose further questions. The interpretation of equivocal outcomes of intervention studies also poses moral responsibilities of the type of 'acts or omissions', particularly in the case of the possible failure of preventing a potentially preventable mass disease. In behavioural intervention, the risk/benefit ratio may have socio-cultural shades that need to be considered when making ethical judgments. To avoid discourse in a vacuum, all these issues will be discussed, using the example of case histories of selected prevention studies carried out recently in Europe and North America.

Complexity of Ethical Issues in Prevention Studies

The extreme complexity that can be faced in the planning of some prevention trials is illustrated nicely by the first case history. In the mid 1960s it became clear that the theory that high blood lipid levels may cause atherosclerosis had a solid basis, established by descriptive, both cross-sectional and prospective epidemiological studies. It remained to be tested whether an intervention on the lowering of serum lipids in clinically healthy people would prevent coronary heart disease. A primary prevention trial of coronary heart disease was, therefore, set up. Clofibrate was given to a large number of informed volunteers in a double-blind trial, with a control group which was given olive oil as placebo and another control group which was simply observed. Fifteen thousand people were studied for a total of 208 000 observation years.

The results of the trial showed that long-term administration of clofibrate does lower serum cholesterol and reduces the incidence of non fatal coronary heart disease by about 20 per cent. But this beneficial effect of clofibrate was cancelled out by an excess mortality observed in the clofibrate group compared with the group which was receiving olive oil.[16–18]

Was this intervention trial ethically justified or not? It must of course be remembered that, at the time when the trial was planned and started, clofibrate was considered a harmless chemical with no known side-effect. There was also much less concern about the ethics of such research than there is today.

Analysis of the justification of the trial produces several positives and several negatives. From the modern viewpoint, the trial was not justified ecologically. Moderately elevated serum lipids can be lowered by natural means and there can therefore be no justification for lowering them chemically. The total amount of clofibrate given in this trial over the years amounted to 30 millions grams. If—as it should—the deontological importance of the preservation of the chemical and physical environment is recognized, the trial was not justified, since a considerable quantity of a chemical substance was administered internally to many human subjects.

On the other hand, the trial *was* justified, paradoxically, because of its negative outcome. If the trial had not been carried out, clofibrate would not have been discredited as a means of primary prevention and would have continued to be prescribed over many decades to come in unlimited quantities.

There is another positive in the fact that the study has confirmed the lipid theory of atherogenesis. That was an important scientific gain and contributes to the future of coronary prevention.

Another negative, on the other hand, lies in the fact that, although the trial demonstrated that clofibrate is inappropriate for primary prevention of ischaemic heart disease, the result has simply been a shift in prescribing habits. Doctors started prescribing other drugs from the same family—for example, fenofibrate or bezafibrate—instead. Since these drugs have not been tested with the same rigour as clofibrate, they continue to be prescribed. Looked at from this point of view, the trial has merely had a superficial effect on prescribing and this introduces the complex issue of implementation of results. A recent analysis of the impact of controlled trials on the progress of therapy in cardiovascular diseases[10] suggests that the mere performance of trials may fail to modify prescribing habits. At any rate, it is important to assess the effects of such trials on actual medical practice and behaviour. We may hope that in the long run the trial will contribute to the reshaping of prescribing habits. This kind of analysis or 'autopsy' highlights the complexity of the ethical issues involved in such a trial. The difficulty, however, is that it is virtually impossible to foresee all such contradictory issues when planning and seeking approval for this kind of research.

Informed Consent in Population Studies

This problem of informed consent has been reviewed elsewhere[3] but it may be useful in the present context to look at the issue with a precise example. In the mid 1970s, it became evident that community programmes for the control of different chronic diseases often overlap to a considerable extent and that their efficiency could be enhanced by integrating several single disease programmes into a more comprehensive action. The World Health Organization undertook therefore to verify the feasibility and assess the effects of comprehensive cardiovascular control programmes and offered a study protocol to a number of countries ready to participate in a cooperative study. Comprehensive intervention including public information and education, continuing education of health professionals and reorganization of health services was to be established in study communities, matched by 'reference' communities without such programmes.

In country Y, the council of city N (150 000 inhabitants) was informed about the protocol and unanimously agreed on behalf of the community, to build up an intervention programme. The request to act as a 'reference' community was refused, however, by city council S (110 000 inhabitants) with the (verbal) explanation: 'We don't play guinea pigs'.

In both instances, the city councils considered that acceptance or refusal was within their own competence, without consulting the population at large. Yet, acceptance of the programme by council N implied, among other inconveniences, taking blood samples from many citizens (although, of course, this still could be individually refused). On the other hand, refusal by council S implied depriving their citizens of the potential benefits of improved health statistics and analyses of health care. Since there was no precedent of this kind, it is unlikely that the city councils could have been mandated specifically for taking a decision in such a matter. The somewhat theoretical bio-ethical question is, was the team of investigators morally right in accepting the decision of the city councils instead of seeking the opinion of the population that, in theory, could have been obtained by a poll?

The problem of community consent and its surrogates has been reviewed elsewhere.[3] It is sufficient here to emphasize the extremely difficult question of relationships between locally (nationally) prevailing socio-cultural norms and political systems (degrees or directness of democracy), and the perceived ethical attributes of this type of decision-taking. However, even in the 'best of all possible worlds', the conflict between public health and individual liberty[19] cannot be avoided. As in many other fields, there will always be minority interests which will have to be overruled by majority options. Of course, the practical problem is to find out where the majority is. The theoretical argument of 'Kantian' or deontological versus utilitarian ethics is discussed fully by Karhausen in Chapter 3 of this book.

Ethical Questions Related to Age

Studies in children and in the elderly carry some ethical nuances. The ethical considerations on intervention studies in children and adolescents have been reviewed previously,[2] as have the general question of ethics in paediatric medicine.[20] The same remains to be done for the elderly population. Although in a different way and to a different extent, old people share with children the fact that they are a vulnerable and more medically dependent group; when living in homes for the elderly, they may even be a 'captive' population. Nevertheless, the important paediatric problems of eligibility, rights, informed consent and protection[3] apply only marginally or not at all in old age. What is common for both groups is the need for special considerations of the extent of intervention beneficence. Two examples may help to illustrate this problem.

It is generally accepted that blood lipid levels at present observed in children (in developed countries) are far above those considered optimal.[21] Would nutritional intervention in children be ethically justified if we consider that the child as a child will derive no direct benefit from such an intervention, but that it may mitigate the probability of coronary thrombosis in, say, the sixth or seventh decade of his or her life? The perception of remote benefits is discounted in time. A study of the feasibility of such intervention may be started only if the intervention itself is deemed to be ethically justified.

At the other end of the scale would be the example of antismoking intervention in elderly smokers. It never seems too late for prevention,[22,23] but the potential benefits necessarily decrease with the shortening of the remaining life expectancy. On the other hand, smoking cessation and other behavioural changes may require greater efforts in elderly persons with deeply engrained habits.[24] They may be paying more heavily for a shorter lasting benefit than younger people. Especially in the elderly, quality of life should be taken in account when assessing the cost/benefit ratio of a behavioural intervention. Although the concept of quality of life seems to be elusive, there are a number of methods available for its assessment.[25]

In conclusion, when judging the ethical justification of preventive intervention by estimating its beneficence, the age of the individual or group should be considered, although for different reasons, in the young and in the old.

Responsibility in Interpreting Results of Prevention Studies

In the early 1970s, it became evident, again on the basis of descriptive epidemiological studies, that coronary heart disease was associated with multiple risk factors. It remained to be shown that intervention on those risk factors would reduce the incidence of coronary heart disease.

A well designed but expensive trial was carried out over six years on 12 866 high risk, but clinically healthy, individuals, randomized into an intensive intervention group and a control group merely observed. The trial ended recently[26] with a modest result: both the reduction of risk factors and the reduction in disease incidence were less than expected, and the confidence limits of statistical significance were so wide that they did not allow the conclusion that disease incidence was reduced as a result of the intervention. Three interpretations are, therefore, possible: no effect; effect positive in selected subgroups; effect positive but not demonstrable because of certain confounding negative factors.

Scientifically, all three interpretations are valid; which one to choose becomes a matter of judgment. The ethical element comes with the realization of the responsibility attached to the choice of interpretation. The public health issue at stake is enormous. It concerns the definition of health policies and recommendations for hundreds of thousands or millions of people, and raises the question of a possible failure of preventing a possibly preventable mass disease. In terms of utilitarian ethics, the use of any of the above interpretations contains an ethical element—by emphasizing one or the other interpretation, the current movement to prevent coronary heart disease can be hampered or promoted. In all fairness, it should be added that a positive interpretation is facilitated, if this trial is considered in conjunction with three other similar studies.[27] This is to underline the moral responsibility of interpreting equivocal results in the light of *all* available knowledge on the subject, instead of considering only selected information.

Socio-Cultural Values and the Principle of Beneficence

Intervention studies are also a sociological category insofar as they touch on social phenomena. Ethical considerations of preventive studies must not ignore the implications of behavioural intervention for society as a whole.

The case history of a cardiovascular intervention study in the Swiss city of Nyon[28] can serve as an example here. In this town of around 15 000 inhabitants, the feasibility of a coronary risk factor intervention was tested on the entire population. The intervention resulted in certain behavioural changes; the results were compared with the 'spontaneous' changes observed in the town of Vevey, the reference community.

The ethical justification of the study has been challenged recently by a sociological analysis.[29] Besides the customary charges of medicalizing society,[30] transforming healthy people into patients for the sake of financial benefits as, for example, in George Bernard Shaw's *The Doctor's Dilemma*, and Jules Romains's *Le docteur Knock ou la puissance de la médecine* and 'manipulation of the masses in their own interest', the analysis raises the valid question of social class-bound values. Indeed, rich food, smoking and drinking are traditional accompaniments, even mediators, of conviviality and an imposed change in this behaviour may be perceived as a serious loss, unless substituted by other pleasures of life.

An intervention study may thus impinge on the principle of beneficence, unless the benefit exceeds the loss. But how do we measure the loss? As it happens, these risky 'pleasures' require relatively little money and no mental effort. Higher social classes may find it easier therefore to refrain from them than working class people whose quality of life may be jeopardized by forceful, evangelistic health propaganda.[29]

There is little doubt that preventive intervention and, for that matter, any health intervention, should be adapted to the relevant socio-cultural setting. Ways should also be sought not to impair the perceived quality of life of the individuals exposed to intervention, nor to make them feel guilty because of their risky habits. Whenever possible, substitutes should be offered. This should be done for ethical reasons, but also for practical purposes, since simple moralizing or prohibition simply do not work, as shown by the example of prohibition by legislation. These problems are, however, mainly in the domain of methods of health education.

It is true, as documented recently, that when individuals who were feeling well, are labelled as being at high risk, for example, because of arterial hypertension, their quality of life suffers.[31,32] This poses the ethical dilemma, of whether such persons should be told the truth, or whether risk factors (blood pressure) should be assessed at all in the clinically healthy. The arguments need to be considered carefully, but the reasons for an active preventive attitude prevail.[33]

SOME CENTRAL ISSUES IN THE ETHICS OF PREVENTION AND ITS STUDY

The examples of ethical problems discussed above were cases of special dilemmas encountered in the practice of prevention studies. In the background, there are some underlying, central ethical issues which have been discussed throughout this book and which are pertinent to the whole field of preventive medicine. Among these are the conflict between individual autonomy and public interest; the value of health; and the commitment to prevention.

The problem of disparity between community and individual interest recurs whenever a collective preventive measure is being studied or applied. It is an expression of the division between utilitarian and Kantian ethics and is dealt with in Chapter 3.

The concept that health is of value to human beings underlies all ethical considerations in preventive medicine. But of how much value is it? Sociologists contend—and commonplace observations on risky behaviour seem to confirm—that people value health less than the medical profession is inclined to assume. Health does not seem to be particularly important[34] to healthy people and to society, composed as it fortunately is of a healthy majority. But there is a paradox here, so obvious that it would be embarrassing to refer to it, were it not the source of continuing and severe misunderstandings—health is valued only when it is lost. Health, physical health, a trivial category to the healthy, becomes a central value for the sick.

The medical profession is exposed incessantly to a close-up view of illness—the other side of the coin unseen by the majority of the public. Medical people, therefore, feel they have the moral right to insist on the value of health. They—at least those in preventive medicine—also feel it is their moral obligation to insist on the value of health and to promote preventive measures and their studies—much to the displeasure of those (including some sociologists) who perceive and brand such attitudes as paternalism, evangelism or medicalization. The fact that our health care system is in crisis[35] obviously does not detract from the value of health itself. These considerations remain valid when health is given a wider meaning in the sense of the World Health Organization definition of physical, mental and social wellbeing; this implies then that the pursuit of health and, in the present context, the study and pursuit of prevention, should swell the ranks with a variety of other disciplines—as, in fact, it does.

Disease prevention is certainly more than medicine; it calls for a 'new paradigm' of health care,[35] but—with the force of a deontological imperative—it calls also for increasing medical engagement.

REFERENCES

1. MacMahon, B. and Pugh, Th. F. *Epidemiology: Principles and Methods*. Boston: Little Brown, 1970.
2. Jeanneret, O. and Raymond, L. Medical ethics and experimental epidemiology. Considerations and intervention studies in children and adolescents. *Rev Epidemiol Santé Publique* 1978; **26**: 479–499.
3. Jeanneret, O. Ethical aspects of epidemiological research. **In**: Bankowski, Z. and Howard-Jones, N. (eds). *Human Experimentation and Medical Ethics*. Geneva: Council for International Organization of Medical Sciences, 1982.
4. Jeanneret, O. and Raymond, L. Aspects éthiques des études d'intervention. *Rev Epidemiol Santé Publique 1981*; **29**: 269–279.
5. Helmchen, H. and Müller-Oexlinghausen, B. The inherent paradox in clinical trials in psychiatry. *J Med Ethics* 1975; **1**: 168–173.
6. Wing, J. K. The ethics of clinical trials. *J Med Ethics* 1983; **9**: 59–60.
7. Pappworth, M. H. *Human Guinea Pigs*. Harmondsworth: Pelican, 1969.
8. Vere, D. W. Problems in controlled trials—a critical response. *J Med Ethics* 1983; **9**: 85–89.

9. Brett, A. S. Ethical issues in risk factor intervention. *Am J Med* 1984; **76**: 557–561.
10. Boissel, J. P. Impact of randomized controlled trials on the progress of therapy in cardiovascular diseases. *Rev Epidemiol Santé Publique* 1984; **32**: 212–218.
11. Bulpitt, C. J. *Randomized Controlled Clinical Trials*. The Hague: Martinus Nijhoff, 1983.
12. Editorial: Les essais thérapeutiques en question? *Schweiz Aerztezeit* 1984, **11**: 2282.
13. Marquis, D. Leaving Therapy to Chance. Washington DC: The Hastings Center Report, 1983.
14. Epstein, F. H. The future of long term intervention and prevention studies—methodological aspects. Proceedings of the Fifth International Meeting of Pharmaceutical Physicians. Munich, 14–15 October 1984 (in press).
15. *The Belmont Report. Ethical Principles and Guidelines for the Protection of Human Subjects of Research*. OPRR Reports. Washington DC: US Government Printing Office, 1979.
16. Committee of Principal Investigators. A cooperative trial in the prevention of ischaemic heart disease using clofibrate. *Br Heart J* 1978; **40**: 10691118.
17. Committee of Principal Investigators. WHO Cooperative trial on primary prevention of ischaemic heart disease using clofibrate to lower serum cholesterol: mortality follow-up. *Lancet* 1980; **2**: 379–385.
18. Committee of Principal Investigators. WHO cooperative trial on primary prevention of ischaemic heart disease with clofibrate to lower serum cholesterol: final mortality follow-up. *Lancet* 1984; 600–604.
19. Beauchamp, D. E. Public health and individual liberty. *Am Rev Public Health* 1980; **1**: 121–136.
20. Rochon, J. Ethique et prévention primaire et secondaire. **In**: Royer, P. and Guignard, J. (eds). *Ethique et Pédiatrie*. Paris: Flammarion, 1982.
21. Summary and recommendations of the Conference on blood lipids in children: Optimal levels for early prevention of coronary artery disease. *Prev Med* 1983; **12**: 728–740.
22. Epstein, F. H. Is there an age limit to the prevention of coronary heart disease? *Giornale della Arterosclerosi* 1983; **1**: 30–38.
23. Barrett-Connor, E., Suarez, L., Kay-Tee Khaw, Criqui, M. H. and Wingard, D. L. Ischemic heart disease risk factors after age 50. *J Chron Dis* 1984; **37**: 903–908.
24. Strasser, T. (ed). *Cardiovascular Care of the Elderly*. Geneva: World Health Organization, (in press).
25. Wenger, N. K., Mattson, M. E., Furberg, C. D. and Elinson, J. (eds). Assessment of quality of life in clinical trials of cardiovascular therapies. New York: Le Jacq, 1984.
26. Multiple risk factor intervention trial research group: multiple risk factor intervention trial. Risk factor changes and mortality results. *JAMA* 1982; **248**: 1465–1477.
27. Richard, J. L. Les essais de prévention primaire multifactorielle des cardiopathies ischémiques. *Rev Epidemiol Santé Publique* 1985; **33**: 121–133.
28. Groupe d'étude du Programme National de Recherche no 1. *Prévention des Maladies Cardio-vasculaires en Suisse*. St Saphorin: Georgi, 1982.
29. Gillioz, L. La prévention comme normalisation culturelle. *Schweiz Zeit Sociol* 1984; **1**: 37–84.
30. Illich, I. *Medical Nemesis: The Expropriation of Health*. London: Calder and Boyars, 1974.
31. MacDonald, L. A., Sackett, D. L., Haynes, R. B. and Taylor, D. W. Labelling in hypertension: a review of the behavioural and psychological consequences. *J Chron Dis* 1984; **37**: 933–42.
32. Milne, B. J., Logan, A. G. and Lanagan, P. T. F. Alterations in health perception and life-style in treated hypertensives. *J Chron Dis* 1985; **38**: 37–45.

33. Strasser, T. Results of mild hypertension trials: a synthetic view. **In**: Hoffman, A., Schrey, A. (eds.) *Control of Hypertension in the Prevention of Cardiovascular Disease*. Stuttgart and New York: Schattauer Verlag, 1986.
34. Buchmann, M., Karrer, D. and Meier, R. *Der Umgang mit Gesundheit und Krankheit im Alltag*. Berne: Paul Haupt, 1985.
35. Grémy, F. Will our health system fall apart? The need for a new paradigm. *Effective Health Care* 1984; **1**: 239–247.

Ethical Dilemmas in Health Promotion
Edited by S. Doxiadis

CHAPTER 16

Organization of Ethical Control

JEAN MARTIN

SUMMARY

As one deals with ethical control in the implementation of preventive programmes in whole communities, the issues involved are rather different from those in research and curative medicine. This has to do with the varying nature of the contract between provider and beneficiary of services, with the fact that target groups are, at least subjectively, not ill, and with the impracticability of always obtaining explicit consent. As compared with person-orientated research or care, ethical control in prevention is closer to the ways in which the community tries to resolve issues of general interest. Participation from the public or from some legitimate representatives is required. In this regard, the provision of relevant, understandable and sufficient information is a major requirement and a difficult one to meet. Three major types of preventive action have to be considered and I will look at each of these in turn: (1) health protection or passive primary prevention; (2) large-scale active primary prevention or health promotion. (3) individual preventive measures. The establishment of Ethical Committees and their structure is also discussed in detail along with the whole question of ethical supervision and control, and practical examples are given.

ETHICAL CONTROL IN PREVENTIVE PRACTICE

In this chapter I will deal with control in practical actions and programmes carried out generally in the community. These situations are rather different from those in which ethics have mostly been discussed, that is, research[1-3] and clinical care,[4,5] where in the last 15 years review procedures have gradually become routine.

Biomedical research centred on individual people or patients usually differs from its preventive counterpart in the following ways: it is carried out usually in university or industrial settings which are comparatively rare and well defined;

the number of subjects is usually limited—a few tens or a few hundreds—and a personal relationship between them and the researcher exists or can be built up.

As compared with clinical work in therapeutic medicine, there are several characteristics of prevention which make ethical control different in this context. These were described by Doxiadis in his Introduction to the book and I will reiterate them briefly here. The relationship, the contract, between recipient and provider of service is not identical. It is usually less well defined in preventive work and it is not always clear that the recipient has given a mandate to the provider. Recipients are usually healthy people, at least subjectively, they do not come with a health complaint and therefore might well be less ready to accept any action suggested, even when this is intended to promote their wellbeing. Prevention also shows its beneficial effects only in the mid or long term. In prevention, one often deals with *groups* of people instead of one or a few in clinical work. This can make it difficult to obtain specific informed consent from all those concerned.

In discussing ethical control in prevention, I shall refer to situations where the biomedical or natural science aspects of the case are known to our satisfaction—it is certain, for example, that iodization of table salt prevents endemic goitre; it has been scientifically shown that smoking is a very strong risk factor as regards the development of lung and other cancers; it is generally accepted that the number of severe injuries and deaths that can be prevented by the compulsory use of seat-belts in cars is very much higher than the rare problems possibly caused by the belts. However, even when the preventive potential of a measure is known, its implementation requires to be accompanied by an evaluation in the community. As Dunne[6] says:

> 'Wherever interventionist public health policies are accepted as a function of government, a complementary need to assess and to monitor the consequences of such measures from the time they are planned—and for as long as they remain in operation—must be accepted, not only by the responsible authorities, but by the community at large.'

The questions discussed below, therefore, focus on the need to ensure there is sufficient ethical appreciation in the relevant country or community of the acceptability and appropriateness of proposed or existing preventive measures.

ETHICAL CONTROL AND VARIOUS DIMENSIONS OF PREVENTION

It is important to examine how the ethical situation varies according to the types or facets of prevention involved.

Primary, Secondary and Tertiary Prevention

By definition, in primary prevention, the disease is not yet present, and in most cases one cannot say whether, without prevention, it would certainly occur in the future. In secondary prevention, one looks for already existing disease, at an early stage more amenable to effective treatment. This is, therefore, closer to the position in curative medicine as is tertiary prevention involving rehabilitation after illness or accident.

Prevention Under Public or Private Auspices

In many countries, private organizations play an important role in preventive activities, particularly in health education and promotion. As private groups have no legal power they can bring to bear on citizens, the ethical risks involved would therefore be smaller than when the public authority is taking charge. This does not mean, let me emphasize, that it is not appropriate for the State to engage in prevention! Frequently, however, such private organizations receive significant state support and this can obscure or lessen the difference between the public and private sectors.

Health Benefit from the Proposed Preventive Action

Preventive medicine specialists and others insist more and more on the necessity of weighing carefully, in assessing the potential of prevention programmes, the likely health benefits and the various costs involved—financial costs, social costs, administrative control and registration and so on. This has relevance as well for ethical aspects.

THREE MAIN AREAS OF PREVENTION

In practice, there are three main areas to which most preventive actions can be related.

The first of these can be described as *health protection* or '*passive*' *primary prevention*. This refers to measures which, once decided upon in principle, are usually applied on a long-term basis by the public authority, without the individual citizen having influence on them and with time often without the individual even being aware of them. Examples of this are iodization, fluoridation of drinking water (or, as is the case in Switzerland, of table salt); legislation about water treatment, control of foodstuffs and other products in common use, as well as of medical drugs; speed limits, obligatory use of restraints in traffic, and other regulations in this field; mandatory immunizations; regulations aiming at the protection of the environment (about land use, building, industrial development, pollution).

The second area of activity can be described as *health promotion* or '*active' primary prevention* in the whole community or for large groups. These are programmes with a large health education component, based in the community, and trying to promote behaviour changes and new life-styles among the population. The health problems such activities are aimed towards include cardiovascular disease, smoking, alcohol abuse, unfavourable nutritional habits, lack of physical exercise, dangerous driving.

The major ethical question in this area concerns the prevention–individual freedom interface, the question of paternalism versus autonomy, fully discussed in relation to the alcohol problems in Chapter 7. To what extent is it acceptable to influence or force people's actions even when it is for their own good?[7,8]

The third area of preventive activity can be described as *individual prevention* or *prevention in personal health care*. In the practices of physicians or other health professionals, preventive activities are directed to individuals or small groups. Examples here include health promotion and active primary prevention as mentioned above and although such activities within personal care are not yet common, there is an agreement that care providers should develop this area; and more frequently secondary prevention procedures such as Papanicolaou smear, breast examination for tumour, detection of latent or early diabetes, elevated blood pressure, and so on.

In what follows I shall refer particularly to the health protection/passive prevention activity. This is the area which raises ethical questions most often, since it is characterized by intentions or acts of the State with the aim of protecting citizens without their active involvement.[9] But the same general principles remain valid for all preventive situations and it is easy to see how what applies to health protection can be adapted to fit the other types of activity. The significant difference is that the latter imply less public constraint—the person or patient concerned can exercise his own will not only when the initial decision is taken (which might be the case for health protection measures), but at any time. Even in large-scale health education programmes, the issue can be then one of paternalism, but there is no obligation to behave healthily.

In individual-orientated prevention (especially secondary prevention), there is a patient–provider relationship comparable to what exists for health care in general. As regards ethics, prevention carried out under those auspices can often be assimilated to clinical care. It is provided in the same form, within the same contract between professional and care-requesting person or small group. Further, the consulting person often does not make, in these conditions, a clear difference between care with a preventive objective and care for curative purposes.

It is important as well that the consulting person is free to change care provider if he or she is unsatisfied with the attention received. This represents a protection, although of course it is quite difficult for patients to evaluate the relevance and the quality of the service they receive. This makes it appropriate and necessary for the physician or other health professional to observe in prevention the same ethical principles he would observe in curative work.

THE ISSUE OF INFORMED CONSENT

When it is proposed to introduce collective measures to protect or promote the health of the public or of large groups, how is the agreement of those subjected to the measure to be obtained? It might be impracticable, and certainly very burdensome, to have to reach hundreds of thousands of people. There may also be a risk of misunderstanding or a distortion of the reasons why such a formal procedure—such as asking for a signature—is required. This might, for example, lead to an exaggeration of the risk potentialities of the programme. For aspects of clinical research, there are currently, in Continental Europe at any rate, professional people and even ethical review committees who think that it is sometimes inappropriate to require written consent, especially in view of prevailing attitudes and socio-cultural contexts[10] but the situation is changing relatively slowly.

On issues that have created controversies—such as iodization and fluoridation, particularly in the United States,[11] or obligatory use of restraints when travelling in motor vehicles, as well as speed limits—a form of written consent has been sought through popular votes. In Switzerland, the seat-belt issue was submitted to the people in 1980 and they decided by a small margin to make the use of seat-belts obligatory.

More frequently, parliaments are called upon to decide on programmes with a preventive purpose and in practice these decisions are often made without close parliamentary supervision on relevant health protection regulations. We find again here this characteristic of large-scale prevention which makes it very different from the provider–patient relationship usual in other aspects of health care. For ethics to be adequately considered, it is clearly not sufficient for professionals to adopt the appropriate attitudes and practices. Some additional mechanisms, securities, and guarantees are needed.

One possible answer is the creation of Ethical Review Committees at relevant levels and with appropriate power and scope of concern. Several relevant aspects will be discussed below—it will be suggested in particular that such committees should be advisory, that they should not be given the power of decision. Who then takes the ultimate decision as to whether a preventive measure is sufficiently ethical and useful to justify its general implementation in the community?

This raises the question of whether a decision taken by Parliament or by the people is to be considered ethical for the community involved at a given point in time. This is a complex question. In absolute terms, the question can hardly be 'yes'. It is certain that, in the past as today, even decisions taken by due democratic process in Western European and North American countries may be questionable from an ethical point of view. The main risk is that of unfairness to minorities. This makes for especially difficult and unsatisfactory situations when the community is markedly heterogeneous, and when there are clear-cut and rather permanent lines between various groups—when majorities are unlikely to change according to the objective merits of the specific topic, for example, because political agreements and oppositions remain routinely the same among population 'blocks'.

In relative terms, however, where the constitutional and legal framework permits, one should not exclude resort to popular votes or a referendum: for example, when the majority conflicting point is in relation to the prevention–individual freedom conflict. A referendum might be the 'less bad' way to judge whether it is acceptable to impose on a community the fluoridation of its water supply, or an obligation to use seat-belts, or increased taxes on alcohol, or prohibition of some forms of advertising, or specific pollution control measures. But it is essential to ensure that the facts of the case are known and presented fairly beforehand to those who have to decide by means of relevant, sufficient and understandable information. This is a serious challenge which might well not often be met successfully even in programmes aimed at specific groups.[12] Issues concerning health protection should be presented in ethical terms in addition to the biological, medical, economic and other aspects, and not in a partisan political way. Or, rather, they should be presented in terms of politics as *res publica*, as the search for optimal community wellbeing. Experience shows, however, that it is difficult to avoid politicization.

Community-wide referenda are used on occasion in Switzerland, for example. However, similar considerations hold true for the possible role of parliaments in deciding on preventive measures. There also all aspects should be considered and the same care should be taken to ensure that complete, objective information is available to the decision-makers.

ETHICAL REVIEW COMMITTEES

The creation of such committees, called Institutional Review Boards in the United States,[13] is a possibility which readily comes to mind for control purposes. The developments in this respect since the 1970s have been documented and discussed on a global basis and in specific countries.[1-3,14-18]

These boards are often an appropriate instrument. In the past, however, they have been instituted especially in university settings for the supervision of research and aspects of curative care. It is important to accept that, in the case of preventive programmes applied or offered to large numbers of persons, the situation is rather different: ethical committees have then to advise or refer, in one way or another, to the whole community rather than to academic bodies.[19-21] This represents a significant change in emphasis.

Composition of the Committee

The committee should include representatives of the major sectors concerned so that several dimensions are taken into account: medical and health, sociocultural, non-partisan political aspects, and economic factors—when a measure requires the use of significant resources, there is always an ethical debate as to whether those resources might not be better allocated elsewhere. Members will be chosen from among the following groups although this list is not intended to be exhaustive or obligatory: concerned health and social professionals (physicians, nurses, social workers, and so on); political and administrative decision-makers; consumers and users of health services (in some cases, parents of subjects involved); ethicists, religious scholars and priests; sociologists, cultural anthropologists; lawyers, judges; journalists and representatives of the communications field and media.

With regard to economic aspects, it may be appropriate to have a representative of the health insurance and sickness funds sector. The selection of representatives of the public, of consumers and patients, desirable and usually accepted now, presents certain difficulties. It is not always obvious who may be a credible, legitimate delegate in this category.[22] The groups in which one might look for such members include legislators, trade unions, consumer associations, women's organizations, self-help and other organized groups with interests in health and quality of life issues.

Who Appoints the Ethical Review Committee?

This depends on the level and the difficulty of the issues to be dealt with by the committee. In many countries and areas of the world—for example, in Western Europe—the final compromise will probably be that the political power, the concerned level of government should appoint the committee. This level is not always the national one, especially in federal structures—for example, the United States (States), the Federal Republic of Germany (Länder), or Switzerland (Cantons). It should also be clear that several committee members, perhaps most of them, will in fact be proposed by non-governmental bodies, in the context of a consultation process by the responsible government office. Their designation by government is thus more in the nature of a ratification. In Switzerland certainly such methods are used frequently. In the last analysis, government is the institution which has to be responsive to characteristics of all sectors of the community. Other groups, for example academics or the professions, usually have a less broad vision of the problems involved and might in some instances be suspected of pursuing their own objectives and interests. It is possible that a commission from an academic or professional group would be entrusted with certain specific tasks by government.

Principles in Ethical Committee Work

The appointment of a given body by public authority should not mean that it cannot function *independently* from government. The principles under which it is established must include guarantees in this regard. Regarding relevant ethical issues, guidelines exist in several countries. In the United States, the US Public Health Service and the National Commission for the Protection of Human Subjects of Biomedical and Behavioural Research have issued a number of such texts,[13] as has the British Medical Research Council, l'Académie Nationale de Médecine in France, and comparable bodies in other countries. The Swiss Academy of Medical Sciences has also published recommendations on several topics which have received attention.[23] WHO and CIOMS have proposed international guidelines.[24] In areas where no guidelines are available, the committees can be entrusted with the task of making proposals.

Another important aspect is the delineation of the committee's sphere of concern. The ethical dimensions it has to appreciate are to be seen in a broad sense but within certain limits as well: thus, it is not the committee's task to judge the strictly scientific qualities of the situation although this must be documented in the information made available to it. In a similar fashion, in the field of biomedical research, ethical committees are not those which judge the scientific interest of planned projects. In Switzerland recently, a Working Group entrusted with proposing measures for the protection of personal data in medical research warned in this regard that one should not, under the guise of ethical concern, allow an undesirable steering and control of parts of scientific activity which have no direct relationship with personal data protection.

One major question is whether the resolutions taken by an ethical committee should have the value of a decision by the authority. In general, it seems preferable that the committee be advisory—that is, that it should issue *recommendations*. This would preserve its independence and maintain a clearer status and mandate—to give advice on ethics. If its resolutions were to be binding, this could introduce a confusion between its role and that of government; government can indeed, if it so wishes, decide that some opinions of the committee are to be obligatorily enforced.

ROLE OF A NATIONAL PREVENTION COUNCIL/COMMISSION

In most countries, there is agreement that prevention has not received the attention and the opportunities it deserves. In recent years, several Government sponsored papers have documented this need: the well-known Lalonde Report, *A New Perspective on the Health of Canadians*[25] in Canada; *Prevention and Health: Everybody's Business*[26] in the United Kingdom; *Healthy People—the Surgeon General's Report on Health Promotion and Disease Prevention*[27] in the United States; *Propositions pour une politique de prévention*[28] in France.

In particular, it has been noted that, in order to give prevention its rightful place, one useful measure (though by no means a panacea) would be to create at a high level a National Council or Committee or Conference on Prevention with a clear mandate to elaborate recommendations and to stimulate research, as well as large-scale preventive programmes. In Switzerland, such a proposal is currently under consideration.

Assuming the creation of such a national body, one of its logical tasks would be to judge the ethical aspects of projects it sponsors, supports or is otherwise aware of. It could also serve as the ultimate advisor in this respect for any prevention-oriented endeavour. Government would thus be able to base and (if needed) justify its initiatives in this field on competent multidisciplinary advice.

Guidelines For and Coordination with Action at the Local Level

In community-based efforts, leadership at the periphery is needed. Initiative by local reference persons or groups is an important ingredient for success. It has to be recognized, however, that the collaboration of outside specialists (coming from more central bodies) is also required. This is true for ethical aspects as it is, for example, for scientific ones.

It is thus desirable that guidelines be developed by a National or Regional Council or Committee which can be made available to local steering groups of preventive programmes. This can help in avoiding errors as a result of insufficient knowledge or experience or repetition of similar projects in a number of different programme sites. Coordination should be ensured so that, while safeguarding the flexibility of local programmes, an appropriate general framework and sufficient coherence can be maintained in a given country or region.

Formal and Informal Control Within the Community

In programmes in the field of active primary prevention with a strong health education component, I mentioned earlier that the main ethical issue concerns paternalism. Sometimes, preventive efforts are labelled cultural or intellectual imperialism and certain concepts are seen as elitist.

It should be underlined that such programmes are voluntary in essence: people are offered opportunities conducive to better health through appropriate life-styles, but remain basically free to choose. To be implemented successfully, it has been clearly shown that these programmes need *effective participation* by many members of the community, who must be involved in the decisions concerning them, from the conception and design stage onwards.[29] Such individuals will be on the local programme committee responsible for running, or at least supervising, all activities. Such a board may include, or at least work closely with, technical experts. And, because of its multidisciplinary composition, it will be in a strong position to judge ethical questions.

One can count on a measure of *informal control* by the community itself. No programme can succeed if it runs harshly counter to prevailing attitudes and practices. In our conditions, the risks of 'moral tyranny' by prevention advocates are slim indeed: any attempt to impose new ways of behaviours on unreceptive people will result in rejection of or indifference to the programme. In a community-based action-research project aiming at prevention of cardiovascular diseases, for example, financed by the Swiss National Science Foundation, it was found in the French speaking part of Switzerland (project site was the town of Nyon) that efforts focussing *directly* on smoking cessation were not well accepted and very few people registered for such activities.[29] In the same area, a vineyard region where wine is very much part of the social mores, little would be achieved by frontal attacks on wine drinking, and alcohol-related health education has to take this factor into account. The same is true for nutritional education. Any authoritarian programme would be discredited before it even began to make an impact.

The main elements of the preceding sections in respect to level and type of ethical control, as well as the related functions of a National Prevention Council, are summarized in Table 1.

THE ISSUE OF BUREAUCRACY/RIGIDITY

There is a current concern about several questions related to ethics. With the original aim of protecting personal dignity and privacy, there has been a tendency to institute cumbersome control procedures without adequate clarification of their effectiveness. It is important to make sure that any control imposed on the activities and discretion of a professional group—for example, the physicians—does not simply transfer the power to another limited influential group, such as lawyers, or administrators or economists, but that it really means increased multisectoral debate and decision-making.

Administrative control procedures are indispensable. But one should not neglect the potential for trust among the interest groups involved and for some reliance on the opinion of recognized 'wise persons' in the community. While circumstances in this respect vary greatly from one socio-cultural context to another, there are in all societies and in all professional groups people who are respected for their knowledge and sound judgment.

Rothman[30] has described (and prophesied!) what the consequences of bureaucratic ethical protection measures can be. One way to minimize them is to avoid taking hasty decisions because the issues are fashionable and there is public pressure, but to consider and weigh carefully the possible side-effects of various systems, in the sense of a broadly based cost–benefit analysis. Controls on the use of personal data, especially from data banks, is a problem which currently excites much discussion and has great influence on progress in preventive medicine and epidemiology. There is already in some countries

Table 1 Ethical control—different procedures and levels for different preventive actions.*

Type of Prevention	Level of control mostly concerned	Major control bodies/procedures	Complementary role by National Prevention Council/Commission (or similar body)
●Health protection 'Passive' primary prevention	National/State	National Prevention Council Parliament/Popular vote	Elaborating and forwarding proposals
●Active primary prevention (health education—health promotion) Community programmes Programmes in organized settings (School, workplace)	Local (community, school or firm concerned)	Programme Committee(s) (Multidisciplinary—including consumers)	Formulating guidelines/concepts recommendations
●Secondary prevention screening *In personal care* (physicians' offices and so on)	'Diffuse' (peer interaction and control continuing education)	Ethical Committees Professional Associations, Specialist Societies, PSRO schemes	Ethical Supervision (including appeals from other levels)
In collective care School health Occupational health	Level legally reponsible for service	Prevention Council Ethical Committees Parliament/Government (national/local)	

*Tertiary prevention (rehabilitation) is not considered specifically here. The ethical issues it may pose are similar to those in curative and palliative care.

evidence that recently adopted schemes of control are barely manageable and create bureaucratic delays. Although planned with the best intentions, those schemes go beyond what is necessary and practicable in real life.

RELEVANT AND FLEXIBLE PROCEDURES FOR ETHICAL CONTROL

As noted above, there are several dimensions of prevention, with different levels of active involvement of the individual. Their technical characteristics and the ways they are put into practice are diverse as well. When elaborating ethical control schemes, a conceptual framework is useful in selecting adequate and efficient means but avoiding heavy or rigid procedures when a satisfactory result can be obtained otherwise.

This kind of framework is summarized in Table 2. Certain features call for more formalized methods with stricter requirements and structures while others allow more flexibility according to technical and professional considerations. These indications are to be seen as finding place along a continuum, between issues which raise few ethical questions and others which pose serious ones.

The association between 'formalized' and 'multidisciplinary' also has its exceptions. There might be cases where a quite formal procedure is necessary, with a limited professional group in charge. However, in general, the more an issue raises ethical problems the more it appears that the control shall be formalized and of an interdisciplinary nature.

ETHICAL APPRECIATION AND CONTROL: EXAMPLES OF CHANGING SITUATIONS

Immunizations

For decades, it has been considered ethically acceptable that smallpox vaccination be required for entire populations although there were instances of severe complications and sometimes death. But the protection of the community at large was considered to prevail over those accidents affecting individuals. The situation has changed radically with the successful eradication of the disease through the programme set up by the World Health Organization and its Member States, attested in 1980. In most countries it would be considered quite unethical today to give (and a fortiori impose) this vaccination.

Other immunizations have entered public discussion, most notably the one against whooping cough in Great Britain. The controversy, which is discussed by Rayner in Chapter 17 of this book, brought a large reduction in the number of children protected and some unfavourable consequences for child health from a community point of view.

Tetanus immunization raises a different point, similar to the one much discussed about the obligatory use of seat-belts. Typically, people not protected

Table 2 What kind of ethical control for what kind of issue?

	The appropriate control procedure is likely to be	
	More multidisciplinary/ participative more formalized	⟷ More technical/ professional less formalized
	According to the following characteristics	
Health problem in the community	A major programme is envisaged for a health problem of limited importance*	Concerned health problem is severe/urgent*
	Sensitive political or religious/ moral issue	Straightforward, non-controversial topic
Preventive measure	(Might be) imposed	Voluntary
	Involving all the community	Involving only limited risk groups
	(Still) debatable health benefit	Clear health benefit
	Still at an experimental stage	Well tried and found safe
	Invasive re physical integrity	Non-physically invasive
	Invasive re privacy (related to sensitive personal characteristics)	Does not threaten privacy
	Complex	Simple, easy to perform
	Difficult to understand by lay people	Easily understandable by the person/patient
	Expensive	Cheap
	Primary prevention (disease not present)	Secondary and tertiary prevention (disease already present)

*This does not imply that severe health problems should be handled in a casual manner. But major, urgent, situations can justify a more directed approach. Conversely, if a health problem is of debatable importance in public or personal health terms, careful scrutiny of ethical and other aspects is the more important before one engages in an action programme.

are taking risks for themselves but they do not endanger others. However, if they do get tetanus, heavy medical expenses have to be supported mainly by the State or through some kind of collective mechanism. Is such 'waste of common resources' acceptable when good protection can be acquired by a safe and cheap measure like immunization (and when other objectives worth pursuing could be attained with the same amount of money)?

Genetics and Prenatal Diagnosis

In recent years, aspects of genetics with significant prevention potential have received much attention. The field of prenatal diagnosis is interesting in that it illustrates the differing importance of the questions touched upon—from very serious ones like detection of hereditary and congenital diseases to others which could be considered trivial, like knowledge of the sex of the fetus in otherwise normal pregnancies. An American research institute has elaborated guidelines in this regard.[31] In Switzerland, a project of alpha-1-fetoprotein screening during pregnancy has given the opportunity to adapt such guidelines to a practical situation.[32] It is worth noting that the latter examples relate mainly to individual oriented secondary prevention. However, the screening measures might be applied to a fairly large group which is not routinely 'requesting' the service.

Environmental Protection

While the progress achieved in communicable diseases makes it less justified in certain cases to impose preventive measures on the population, there is an evolution in the opposite direction in respect to protection of the environment because of the growth of available means of altering our environment and of the increasing use made of these means. It seems clear that the State has to be involved in a major way in this field if we want to avoid grave consequences in the long term. There is thus a need for a strong effort to educate the public, in spite of possible paternalistic connotations, and for norms and mandatory regulations.

Who in this case is going to carry out ethical control? Who is to say how much the freedom of the individual can be limited in order to protect the community? Although it concerns health, this is a field which obviously goes far beyond the medical domain. The control bodies and procedures must therefore belong to many disciplines. In many countries, there is an urgent need for closer collaboration between leaders in health and in environmental protection since these structures have often developed separately in the last two decades. A National Prevention Council, as proposed above, could be an appropriate forum for discussion and elaboration of recommendations for government or parliament.

Battered Persons

This is another problem where prevention is badly needed, with potential for authoritarian measures by the State. In French-speaking Switzerland, public opinion was deeply moved in 1985 by the story of a 6-month old infant, born to a drug-addicted couple, who was so badly beaten that she is now severely handicapped and blind. There is in the region a well-developed medico-social network of professionals who were handling the case but their problem was the ethical one of taking a child away from her addict parents, or leaving the parents the chance that she might be a help in their rehabilitation process. There is often pressure at the present time for more reserve in the use of State power in limiting the rights of citizens. This is clearly an area where multi-disciplinary ethical control in preventive work is needed and difficult.

Other Violence

In a paper on ethics and prevention, Dean Jean Rochon, from the Laval University Medical School, Québec, writes[33]:

> 'Techniques of manipulation and conditioning of human behaviours, applied individually or collectively, are more and more perfected and made more effective . . . Publicity and mass media appear to affect the population's mental health, in relation with problems such as violence and crime. What are the delineations between individual responsibility and the duty of the State to intervene? (p. 99—translated from the French).'

We have no answer to the debate about the role of the media, especially television, in the growth of violence. Yet there are concerns about the level of 'mental pollution', as Jean Hamburger puts it,[34] which we should accept and about whether preventive measures should not be taken for the sake of mental health and balance for example, in youth. Although we do not advocate rigid measures in this respect, the question of some broadly based ethical control mechanism might be relevant.

CONCLUDING COMMENTS

Methods of ethical control in preventive medicine need to be discussed more widely among people responsible for decisions in several sectors. This issue cannot be dealt with uniformly. As it is not concerned with projects taking place essentially in university settings (as research), it has to involve communities and the representatives of various groups within them. Governments and their administrations are involved as they implement health protection measures. Ultimately, parliament and citizens have to take certain decisions in this regard, through the mechanisms (including a referendum when relevant) the community uses for tackling issues in other aspects of life in society.

A substantial debate has to take place on these themes. For that debate to be useful, correct and sufficient information should be available to all sectors concerned, and this represents a challenge.

There is a need for the creation of committees or councils at several levels to supervise ethical aspects of prevention, as well as to propose new measures when appropriate.

Such topics must also be dealt with increasingly in the training of interested professionals.[2] There are many current health problems which call for an interdisciplinary approach, with active communication and collaboration in a team spirit. Yet in the actual training institutions (for example, Faculties of Medicine), the necessary changes are taking place only slowly. Ethical control is one of many themes which demand an evolution which could give practical opportunity for many disciplines to work together.

Finally, it must be remembered that while we must aim at formulating ethical rules and control procedures with wide validity and applicability range, this is not always possible. We are dealing with some absolute values as well as with many which might vary significantly from one country or group to another. In this respect, we draw attention to a statement from a recent meeting about health policy, ethics and human values which, while addressing policy-making, has relevance also for the questions posed by ethical control:

> 'Health policy-making is always, and inescapably, an evaluative task. It is not only that value systems inevitably creep in to bias decision-makers, although they do. It is rather that policy-making logically requires a system of values. In large part those values are determined by culture.[35]'

REFERENCES

1. CIOMS. *Medical experimentation and the protection of human rights*. Howard-Jones, N. and Bankowski, Z. (eds). Geneva: CIOMS, 1979.
2. CIOMS. *Medical ethics and medical education*. Bankowski, Z. and Corvera Bernardelli, J. (eds). Geneva: CIOMS, 1981.
3. CIOMS. *Human experimentation and medical ethics*. Bankowski, Z. and Howard-Jones, N. (eds). Geneva: CIOMS, 1982.
4. Rouzioux, J. M. Les commités d'éthique à l'hôpital. *J Med Legale Droit Med* 1981; **24**: 627–630.
5. Hospital Ethics Committees Surveyed. *Hospitals* 1984; **58**: 52.
6. Dunne, J. F. Ethical review procedures for research involving human subjects. **In**: Bankowski, Z. and Corvera Bernardelli, J. (eds). *Medical ethics and medical education*. Geneva: CIOMS, 1981: 77–103.
7. Faden, R. and Faden, A. (eds). Ethical issues in public health policy: Health education and life-style interventions. *Health Educ Monogr* 1978; **6**: (2).
8. Beauchamp, D. E. Public health and individual liberty. **In**: *Ann Rev Public Health*. Palo Alto: Annual Reviews Inc 1980: 121–136.
9. Martin, J. Potential and limits of health legislation, with particular respect to prevention. **In**: Eimeren, W. V. *et al.* (eds). *Third International Conference on System Science in Health Care*. Berlin-Heidelberg: Springer, 1984: 1267–1271.
10. Curran, W. J. Evolution of formal mechanisms for ethical reviews of clinical research. **In**: Howard-Jones, N. and Bankowski, Z. (eds). *Medical experimentation and the protection of human rights*. Geneva: CIOMS, 1979: 11–20.
11. Crain, R. L., Katz, E. and Rosenthal, D. B. *The politics of community conflict—The fluoridation decision*. Indianpolis and New York: Bobbs Merrill Inc, 1969

12. Farfel, M. R. and Holtzman, N. A. Education, consent and counseling in sickle cell screening programs: report a survey. *Am J Public Health* 1984; **74**: 373–375.
13. National Commission for the Protection of Human Subjects of Biomedical and Behavioral Research. *Institutional review boards*. Publication no (OS) 78-0008. Washington: DHEW, 1978.
14. Levine, R. J. The value and limitation of ethical review committees for clinical research. **In**: Bankowski, Z. and Corvera Bernardelli, J. (eds). *Medical ethics and medical education*. Geneva: CIOMS, 1981, 43–63.
15. Isambert, F. A. De la bio-éthique aux comités d'éthique. *Etudes (Paris)* 1983; 671–683.
16. Mach, R. S. and Gsell, O. La création de commissions d'éthique médicale. *Schweiz Aerztezeit* 1980; **61**: 256–257.
17. André A. L'organisation et le fonctionnement des comités d'éthique en Belgique. *J Med Legale Droit Med* 1981; **24**: 647–653.
18. Institut national de la santé et de la recherche médicale. Le Comité consultatif national d'ethique pour les sciences de la vie et de la santé. Paris: Dossier INSERM (typewritten), 2 décembre 1983.
19. Veatch, L. Community participation in health care decisions. Veatch, R. M. and Branson, R. (eds). *Ethics and Health Policy*. Cambridge, MA: Ballinger, 1976, 289–306.
20. The role of the individual and the community in the research, development, and use of biologicals, with criteria for guidelines: A memorandum. *Bull WHO* 1976; **54**: 645–655.
21. Riis, P. Scope of ethical review. **In**: Bankowski, Z. and Howard-Jones, N. (eds). *Human experimentation and medical ethics*. Geneva: CIOMS, 1982: 226–230.
22. Martin, J. Qui représente les patients? Quelques aspects d'une problématique actuelle. *Soins infirmiers/Krankenpflege* (Berne) 1983, **7**: 54–58. Reprinted in: *Ouvertures (Paris)* 1984; **33**: 20–26.
23. Académie suisse des sciences médicales (Swiss Academy of Medical Sciences). Ethical principles and guidelines (several documents). Petersplatz 13, CH–4051 Basel.
24. WHO/CIOMS. Proposed international guidelines for biomedical research involving human subjects. Geneva, 1982.
25. Lalonde, M. *A new perspective on the health of Canadians*. Ottawa: Government of Canada, April 1974.
26. *Prevention and health: everybody's business*. Department of Health and Social Security. London: HMSO, 1976.
27. *Healthy People—The Surgeons General's Report on Health Promotion and Disease Prevention* (2 vols). US Department of Health, Education and Welfare, DHEW (PHS) Publication no. 79-55071 and 79-55071 A. Washington DC, 1979.
28. *Propositions pour une politique de prévention* (Rapport au Ministre de la santé) Paris: La Documentation Française, 1982.
29. Lehmann, P. Prévention des maladies cardio-vasculaires—methodes d'éducation pour la santé et évaluation (Nyon). *Cah Med Soc (Geneva)* 1983; **27**: 1–157.
30. Rothman, K. J. The rise and fall of epidemiology, 1950–200 AD, *New Engl J Med* 1981; **304**: 600–602.
31. Powledge, T. M. and Fletcher, J. Guidelines for the ethical, social and legal issues in prenatal diagnosis. *N Engl J Med* 1979; **300**: 168–172.
32. Commission d'éthique médicale pour l'étude AFP—Suisse. Prise de position. *Schweiz Aerztezeit* 1981; **62**: 1385–1388.

33. Rochon, J. Ethique et prévention primaire et secondaire. **In**: Royer, P. and Guignard, J. (eds). *Ethique et pédiatrie*. Paris: Flammarion Médecine-Sciences, 1982: 92–106.
34. Hamburger, J. *L'homme et les hommes*. Paris: Flammarion, 1976: 153.
35. Veatch, R. **In**: *Health Policy: Ethics and Human Values—An International Dialogue* (Highlights of the Athens Conference, October-November 1984). Geneva: CIOMS, 1985: 10.

Ethical Dilemmas in Health Promotion
Edited by S. Doxiadis

CHAPTER 17

Mass Communication Media in Health Education

CLAIRE RAYNER

SUMMARY

This chapter deals with the relationship between the media and health education. Problems arising from presentation of health and medical matters in three main media groups are discussed. Attention is drawn to the two-dimensional media approach to preventive medicine or health education—first, and attracting much more public and popular attention, what the health professionals can do for individuals, and secondly what individuals can do for themselves. Specific examples of the effects of mass media coverage of health matters are provided. Finally, the suggestion is made that a centralized reliable source of medical information for journalists from all forms of media would be a practical approach to the current difficulties of communication.

INTRODUCTION

A definition of terms is important to any discussion; it is particularly so when the discussion covers a field which is subject to a great deal of confusion and prejudice—and the uses and values of mass communication media are just such a field.

Take the term 'media' itself; it is a word that means a plural yet it is frequently used by both academics and non-academics as though it were a term which describes a single entity, instead of being what it is—a very loose label for a very large group of very different methods of publication. It is often used as a pejorative term, seeming to carry for many people sinister overtones (the 'media' is seen as exploitative, unscrupulous, totally commercial and so on). The word is particularly likely to be used in this way by medical people, in my experience. Doctors have long fulminated against the malign influence of the media and blamed it for damaging the relationship they have with their patients by providing those patients with information and ideas they should not, in the doctors' opinion, have. Many of them responded to a mention of medicine on television, for example, with a 'spate of letters'[1] and continued to do so over several weeks without any of them ever mentioning the fact that the journal in which they were expressing their distrust or dislike of 'the media' is itself part of that media.

It is possible that the word collected its poor image and meaning because it spilled over into everyday use from advertising, which is regarded by many as a particularly cynical and exploitative sales method (a far from justified view in my opinion although that is not a subject that can be dealt with usefully here). But whatever the source of the word's bad reputation, that reputation does exist. It is, therefore, of great importance to this chapter to provide a clear account of what it is that is being discussed.

There are three main groups that comprise the media—the written word, accompanied or not by printed pictures; the spoken word—that is, radio, audio cassettes, phonograph records; and the spoken word accompanied by pictures, still or moving—that is, television, cinema, videos and so on. Each of these has its subgroups; thus, advertising posters fall into the first group; popular songs fall into the second; live theatre performances fall into the third. It will be useful to consider what is provided by some of the components of each group.

THE MASS COMMUNICATIONS MEDIA

Newspapers provide news, feature material, information, opinion, entertainment, and, of course, advertising, which is a very pervasive and powerful informer and manipulator or both.

Magazines provide the same as newspapers but also fiction, another important method of communicating ideas and information.

Television (in all its manifestations, including cable pay-as-you-view, computer programmes for home use and other semi-closed systems) offers the same mix with the addition of silent visual input which can be extremely powerful; when a popular comedian lights a cigarette in the middle of his act, for example, he is sending out an exceedingly strong message without saying a word. Similarly, the use of alcohol by characters in drama offered as popular entertainment is possibly a trigger to increased use by the audience. A British member of the European Parliament complained in February 1985 about what he regarded as over-use of alcohol in a popular American 'soap-opera' programme, *Dynasty*, and his comments were widely reported, and, it is suggested, have persuaded the producers to reduce the amount of alcohol their characters consume.

Radio offers once again the same mixture as the preceding categories but adds the immediacy of the live 'phone-in' programme in which listeners in interacting with the presenter of the programme add their own store of knowledge (and/or ignorance!) to the station's output. It also offers fiction in the form of drama, and this can be used for medical purposes—when characters in *The Archers* a popular radio serial in Britain—became blood donors, so did a very large number of listeners.

Cinema and *video* may not appear to offer such ingredients of the mix as news and features, opinion and information, but in fact they do. Apart from the dramatized documentary film such as *Champions* which deals with the real life experience of a young jockey suffering from cancer of the testis and which told many people of the disease and its treatment, there is the outright fiction film which contains medical information; the famous scene in *Gone With The Wind* in which a character gives birth in a state of great pain and anguish has probably affected more women's expectation of the childbirth experience than any amount of carefully designed educational material put out by obstetricians and midwives.

The *live theatre* plays an important role too, even although it is experienced by far fewer people than have access to television, cinema and video. Not only is it attended by the people who could be called opinion formers, it also frequently feeds the wider media, especially television and the cinema. An example of the health information content of theatre can be found as far back as Ibsen's *Ghosts* which brought some facts about venereal diseases to the attention of a much wider public than had ever considered the matter before. Such theatrical exploration of medical themes continues today—the comparatively recent Brian Clark play, *Whose Life Is It Anyway?* being an obvious example in Britain.

HEALTH EDUCATION

With this definition of the media offered, it is now necessary to define 'health education'. This can be both positive—that is, techniques used to give people information it is believed they should have and advice on what they should do—and negative, giving people messages it is believed they should *not* have, and directives they should *not* obey. In the latter category comes the use of tobacco and alcohol in popular entertainment as already discussed.

It has also been suggested that a medium itself may provide negative health education. The authors of the book[2] *Health, The Mass Media and the National Health Service* say '. . . a television policy which seeks to maximize audiences is effectively an implicit leisure policy and therefore an implicit health policy since it encourages sitting and watching in preference to other activities.'

Health professionals will have their own definition of what health education is and should be; more useful to this discussion is the general public's definition, and I am able to describe the ways in which it sees the health education content of papers, magazines, television and radio because I am told what it is by the readers/viewers/listeners of the various journals and programmes to which I contribute.[3]

THE PUBLIC VIEW OF HEALTH EDUCATION

The public has a two-pronged view of preventive medicine and health education. There is first what *they* (the health professionals and providers) can do for you and to you, and secondly what *you* can do for yourself.

In the first category comes all that derives from contacts with health professionals at doctors' surgeries, hospitals and clinics. It includes immunization programmes, screening services, and such matters as water fluoridation programmes.

Many people are so fascinated by medical matters in this category that plays, films and stories which are set in and around hospitals and doctors' surgeries seem to have a never ending appeal. A new drama series dealing with the work and experiences of a group of general practitioners is currently building a large television audience in Britain, just as its predecessors *Emergency Ward Ten* and *Dr Kildare* did in the fifties.

The public are equally fascinated by real life medical drama. In the United Kingdom newspapers and magazines as well as television and radio have dealt in great detail recently with such matters as *in vitro* fertilization, organ transplants, the provision of haemodialysis resources for sufferers from kidney disease, the provision of funds for open heart surgery, cancer therapies, the care of Down's Syndrome babies, and the provision of cervical smear services, all arising out of news stories about individual cases. The amount of health information gained from these public discussions cannot be measured, of course, but it is reasonable to suppose it is considerable.

Less fascinating for the public at large seems to be discussion of what an individual can do for himself to promote health—that is, when such matters as the need to control tobacco and alcohol use are publicized. However, there has been in recent years an enormous public interest in dietary and exercise regimes, some of which are, in orthodox medical eyes, far from healthy. The publication of a number of books by actresses who have discovered the addictive nature of over-exercising (they appear to be pushing themselves beyond the pain barrier in order to encourage the secretion of endorphins, an experience they find interesting and satisfying) has created a massive multi-million dollar industry, while any book on diet can, if it is absurd enough (for example, *The Beverly Hills Diet* by Judy Mazel) enjoy huge sales.

Together with this there has been a growing interest in health foods, ranging from bran for the bowels to ginseng for improved sexuality via a range of vitamin and mineral supplements for the health value of which there is scant evidence. However, the lack of scientific proof of any good does not curb people's enthusiasm for self-dosage with such nostra, any more than it has prevented an upsurge of interest in 'fringe' medicine. Herbalists, naturopaths, chiropracters, rolfers, radiobionicists and others have never enjoyed so much popularity. This is indeed the age of the quack, and newspapers and television reflect this interest faithfully, publishing and transmitting a great deal of material on the subject. It is also important to be fair at this point; it is impossible to say whether the upsurge of interest in what has been dubbed 'alternative' medicine is a result of the publication of material about it, or whether the publication is a result of the existing interest. Most experienced editors, writers and journalists maintain that they act as mirrors of public interest, not creators of it, and that failure to produce for consumers what they find of interest is commercial suicide, since they stop buying the publication, or viewing the programme, and it dies. And it has to be said that catering to the lowest level of public taste has made fortunes for many.

Clearly there is in this definition evidence of a conflict between orthodox health care and education based on scientific principles and provided by trained and qualified experts, and non-orthodox care and education provided by others. But the media which publicize and discuss this conflict are not to blame for it; for orthodox medicine to maintain that the media should act as its mouthpiece and never publicize views to which it is in opposition is to ask for a form of censorship.

At this stage, it will be useful to consider some specific examples of the effects of coverage of health matters in mass media.

THE PROBLEMS

Among the most interesting of these problems is the case of pertussis vaccination. In March 1974 a television programme on the safety of pertussis vaccine based on an article published in the *Archives of Diseases in Childhood* appeared.

Three months later the Department of Health and Social Security (DHSS) published its circular CMO 17/74 which advised 'vaccinate'. All through the remainder of the year and into 1975 adverse publicity continued, with special efforts made by one particular newspaper, supported by a Professor of Community Medicine, to campaign against pertussis vaccination although concurrently the Joint Committee on Vaccination and Immunization backed up the DHSS advice.

In June 1976, the prestigious British newspaper, the *Sunday Times*, published a series of articles strongly criticizing the vaccine and advising its readers not to vaccinate, and for the rest of that year there continued to appear, in a number of publications, massive adverse publicity.

By March 1977 the DHSS found it necessary to issue two more circulars (CMO 77/3 and CMO 77/7) deploring the drop in the numbers of vaccinations *against various childhood diseases and not just whooping cough*. In June 1977 the Secretary of State promised compensation for vaccine-damaged children, while the Joint Commitee insisted it was necessary to continue vaccinating. In July 1977 a new epidemic of whooping cough started. In October of 1977 the Ombudsman in his report on Whooping Cough Vaccination condemned the

DHSS for not warning parents earlier of adverse reactions, and the DHSS as a result abandoned a campaign that had been planned to encourage take-up of all vaccinations; not until March 1978 was a campaign launched by the Government to encourage take-up of vaccination, and even then it was a far from strong one. In September 1978 the pertussis epidemic reached a new peak.

In summary, as the result of the widespread publicity—which was at its strongest in one particular newspaper—the rate of immunization for that disease dropped in one year from 80 to 30 per cent and in the ten years since then has only slowly risen again to between 48 and 50 per cent, with an obvious reduction in herd immunity as well as in individual immunity. A mass media campaign, therefore, seems to have resulted in at least 30 or 40 excess deaths of infants from whooping cough in the last decade in the United Kingdom.

Dr Noel Preston, director of the Pertussis Reference Laboratory at Manchester University Medical School said in October 1983, 'Sadly, less than half of our infants are receiving vaccination; parents and their medical advisers are still scared by the mass media though the allegations of brain damage are now known to be utterly false.' And in another paper[4] he wrote, 'If we examine the facts soberly, and if we ignore the fiction and also the hysteria generated by the media, we find that adsorbed pertussis vaccine is now one of the safest and most effective of vaccines. Elimination of whooping-cough, however, depends on the development of herd immunity by the vaccination of at least 80 per cent of the child population. As we are rediscovering, following the widespread rejection of this vaccine, whooping cough can be an alarming, prolonged and sometimes fatal illness. But half-hearted use of the vaccine will have little impact. We know *how* to prevent whooping cough—by giving not less than three doses of adsorbed pertussis vaccine, starting at 3 months of age. The means are available. Have we the will?'

This shortened account of a very important 'argument' between mass media and medicine begs many questions, not least of which is, 'Who is to blame?' Was it all triggered by the activities of one particular Professor of Community Medicine, who pushed his views at one particular newspaper? Or was it the fault of other medical people of equal eminence who did not publicly disagree with him loudly or forcefully enough? Or, was it the fault of the news editors of the newspapers involved who saw the issue just as a 'hot story' and did not think through the possibly damaging effects of such publicity?

Was it the fault of the health educators who failed in the prime task of making certain the public had a thorough understanding of the risks and benefits of pertussis vaccination, and access to reliable advisors? Or was it the family and clinic doctors who were themselves affected by what they read in the mass media (they share newspaper and TV programmes with the laity, after all!) who shared the panic?

And it must be remembered that in the middle of the whole argument, the Ombudsman did throw his weight behind the anti-pertussis vaccine campaign by castigating the DHSS for not warning parents earlier of possible adverse reactions. That clearly fed the news editors' conviction that they were right to publicize the subject in the way they did.

Similar problems have arisen in other medical areas, if not so dramatically as in this example. There is the contraceptive Pill controversy which has raged for over two decades and appears to smoulder on; women have been alarmed, reassured, and then alarmed again, and altogether made thoroughly confused as the arguments for and against the use of this popular method of family planning continue in magazines and newspapers. There have been women who as a direct result of alarming TV programmes abandoned their use of the Pill only to present later with unwanted pregnancies and seeking abortion—a procedure which carries a statistically higher morbidity than Pill usage. There have been women with the much less easy-to-measure problem of cancer phobia triggered by previous use of the Pill; I always have received and continue to receive letters from women who cannot be disabused of the idea that they have doomed themselves to a future painful death because they used the Pill in their youth.

Similarly, there have been media discussions of the pros and cons of hormone replacement therapy (HRT) in the menopause, and many women have over the years suffered great distress from climacteric symptoms and been either enraged because their doctors have refused HRT or alarmed because it had been offered. From my own mail bag it is clear to me that for many women, confidence in the general practitioner's ability to prescribe safely has been sorely eroded as a result of such newspaper and magazine reports; more and more are deeply suspicious of any sort of doctor's prescription, and recent public discussions of the long-term damage that can be done by the misuse of tranquillizers—which many doctors have prescribed heavily over many years—has added to this distrust.

But is this necessarily a bad thing? Some doctors feel it is, preferring a form of medical practice in which the doctor is the one who knows and the patient is the humble suppliant who dips in the fount of the doctor's knowledge. Patients who question are seen as 'bad patients' and the mass media which puts the questions into their heads are seen as the root cause of that badness.

As a medical journalist who has written on many of the subjects here mentioned, and who has encouraged people to collect information and on the basis of that information to question their doctors about what is recommended—(Do I really need a hysterectomy? What is the long-term effect of this drug? What are the possible side effects of this therapy? and so on)—I clearly believe that the informed and questioning patient who can strike up what has been labelled a therapeutic relationship with a doctor is a better served and ultimately healthier patient than one who approaches the practitioner as an ignorant and pliant petitioner. I do know that many doctors—and they are increasing in number—share this view of the 'good' patient and encourage their own patients to be as informed in medical affairs as they can be (often they advise individual patients to write to journalists like me to collect the facts they need!) and are prepared to cope with those who, for whatever reason, manage to collect misleading information and suffer from confusion as a result.

There are also doctors who although they are themselves interested in building good relationships with their patients in which they do offer information, encourage questioning and seek for informed involvement in therapy still feel that medical education should not be given in popular mass circulation publications and programmes. They deny, sometimes vehemently, that they would seek to apply censorship on medical matters—which would, frankly, be virtually impossible in a free society anyway—but they do seek for controls.

But the question again begs to be asked—where does censorship end and control begin? Who is to decide what material should be published and what withheld? Let us take the case of the pertussis vaccine campaign. In the event, the Professor of Community Medicine who expressed his doubts so forcibly and so publicly was wrong; the risk of damage to immunized children turned out to be much less than the risk of damaged to those who were not immunized. But suppose he had been right and his work had uncovered a real area of concern? Would not that campaign then have been seen as beneficial rather than as it now appears, damaging? It is worth remembering that no one took note in time to warn the public in some countries (America was a notable exception) of the dangers of the use of thalidomide in pregnancy.

It is also important to remember that the growth of public interest in what has been labelled fringe or alternative medicine has spawned a number of practitioners who believe that they have something to offer the ailing and that they have the right to display that something to the public gaze. To deny all of them credibility would not help the sick; acupuncture, once dismissed by medical men as mumbo jumbo, is now widely accepted as therapy and osteopaths, once dismissed as mere bone-setters, now enjoy considerable respect from the medical establishment. So, where are controls, if they are to be exercised, to be set? And if you once admit such practitioners as non-medically trained osteopaths and acupuncturists, how can you exclude spiritualists, necromancers and their like who maintain that they too have their successes? Equally one must never forget the placebo effect which works just as well for patients of fringe practitioners as for orthodox ones.

Yet another question remains to be asked; at what point does a system of control on medical publication exercised for benevolent reasons cease to be purely medical and become political? If attempts to control the media today on medical matters succeed, what sort of controls will become more acceptable? Today's control of medical reporting could be tomorrow's control of political reporting and that would be unhealthy for all of us.

There are in any case areas where medicine and socio-political questions merge—an example is the treatment and care of the mentally ill and the criteria used for diagnosis (much Western anxiety has been expressed because some Soviet psychiatrists are seen to be acting as instruments of the State in making their decisions about some dissidents). Other examples include the abortion issue, the treatment of severely damaged neonates and the ethics of *in vitro* fertilization as a remedy for subfertility. Does orthodox medicine wish to forbid discussion of such issues outside their own private media?

THE REMEDY

To obtain answers to these questions while at the same time ensuring that editors and programme makers get the fullest possible picture of the material they are handling and presenting to the wider public, I suggest that practical remedies are needed. It is not enough to say 'Such-and-such should be done' which is the usual answer offered in discussions of this nature. What is required is a system whereby such-and-such can actually *be* done.

The practical remedy I would suggest is a centralized, reliable and, if possible, international information source for all those in need of medical information—journalists, from all forms of media, be they printed or visual or aural, programme producers and even dramatists, remembering the enormous influence exerted by entertainment. The bureau would not be run entirely by doctors—that would give them undue power and therefore ultimately the ability to act as censors—but would include representatives of all the media needing to use medical information, all types of medical practitioner, and also all of those fringe (alternative) disciplines which attract public interest. It would be financed firstly by the media themselves who stand to gain most benefit from the existence of the bureau, by means of regular subscriptions, although offers of financial help from other interested parties could be accepted after careful scrutiny. I am thinking here of pharmaceutical companies; not all of them, despite the bad press they have had from both mass media and learned medical media, are A Bad Thing. They too have much to gain from and much to contribute to public health, and their inclusion in the supporters and users of the bureau would help them as much as it would help the mass media and the medical profession and health educators.

THE ETHICS

One of the first tasks of such a bureau would be to create a basic code of ethics not only for mass communicators but for the health professionals. It is not unheard of for practitioners to manipulate the media to their own ends, after all. It would, I suggest, be rooted in the self-created code of ethics on which most of the medical journalists with whom I have had contact over the 25 years of my involvement in mass media writing and presenting base their professional activities.

We do, to the best of our ability, seek to ensure that we *collect* all the facts available on a subject; *present* them honestly without undue bias from selection;

write as clearly as we can and so ensure that our masters, the editors and programme controllers, are as aware as it is possible for them to be of the truth of what we are saying. If we are blocked by our editors, or attempts are made to coerce us into altering our stories to suit an editorial or proprietorial interest, we *resist*.

I cannot for a moment pretend that we all succeed always in behaving as ethically as we would wish. Under the pressure of deadlines, concern for our own careers, and our own inner beliefs we may, as other people may, stray from our ideals from time to time, but by and large we are not, as is so often suggested, a cynical breed. Most medical journalists—and it is these with which I am most concerned—have a commitment to their speciality which is at least as serious and honest as that held by other workers in the health field, including doctors, nurses and health educators. To suggest that only trained medical personnel—trained, in the accepted sense of that word, to be practitioners rather than commentators—hold ethical values is to be insulting to non-medical people as well as somewhat arrogant. As we must all well know, doctors do not have a monopoly of compassion.

With the aid of existing medical ethical committees there is no reason why a workable ethical code for the production of really valuable health information in mass media should not be created, nor is there any reason why there should not be a similarly workable system for ensuring that busy journalists get what they need as quickly as possible—a sense of urgency is often lacking in doctors when dealing with journalists who have deadlines to meet—and that doctors get what they want, which is honest and accurate reporting.

Many journalists have managed to achieve such systems for themselves; as an individual journalist, I have rarely had any difficulty in persuading eminent medical people to talk to me, and have always met with appreciation of the fact that I always send my copy to those I have interviewed for any correction of error that may be needed. I do not change opinion, of course. As a journalist I am entitled to say what I wish *as long as it is clearly marked as my opinion*, what is unforgiveable in a journalist is to present opinion as fact, and my own method of accounting for my copy to those interviewed as well as to my editor has protected me from falling into that trap.

THE VALUE

I believe firmly that the creation of such a bureau as I have suggested as an information source for all journalists, dramatists, and producers in need of medical guidance, which would be freely available to all comers, and would ensure access to all the best sources of informed opinion, would be of great value to doctors as well as to the public. At present there is an attitude of suspicion on the part of many doctors against mass media communicators who may approach them for information and opinion. Attempts to obtain the best and most reliable guidance are often thwarted by doctors' closing of ranks and refusal to talk to journalists, especially on such delicate issues as transplant surgery, hormone replacement therapy, *in vitro* fertilization and other subjects intensely interesting and relevant to the public. This is an attitude which results in poor or inadequate information being published because editors *will* publish something on these fascinating matters, no matter how hard doctors may try to block them and will use the efforts of non-specialist and therefore less reliable journalists in order to do so, if necessary.

If this information bureau were to exist it could go far towards ensuring that doctors were protected from what they seem most greatly to fear—that is, misrepresentation from ignorance or honest error—and it would also help them to understand the problems the mass media communicator faces in presenting his or her material. The journalists would have the assurance of knowing that the information they obtained was the most accurate available, and more likely to be of benefit than harm to their readers.

Sanctions could be applied to deal with bad journalists; access to the bureau could be denied, and good editors would rapidly learn to accept copy only from people who *did* report honestly and fairly. The point must be made that no power on this earth will ever prevent bad publishers and editors from publishing bad information if it sells; there is no way of controlling, for example, the *National Enquirer* in the United States which has a singularly unfortunate approach to 'medical' stories. But all the same, with this sort of system, I believe and hope, the need for censorship would vanish. Goodwill and active cooperation must surely be of greater effect in this field than controls. With that advantage mass media journals could be more effective health educators than they already are. And few will deny, surely, that a great deal of good has been done in the field of health education by popular journalism and entertainment. It is the earnest wish of a great many workers in this field—and I am one of them—that we do even more. With the help of the doctors and their colleagues, we could.

REFERENCES

1. Series of letters. *Br Med J* 1978—25 February, 503–505; 18 March, 667, 713–716; 8 April, 917–918; 13 May.
2. Best, G., Dennis, J. and Draper, P. *Health—The Mass Media and the National Health Service*. London: Unit for the Study of Health Policy, Department of Community Medicine, Guy's Hospital Medical School, 1977.
3. *Sunday Mirror*—British newspaper with readership estimated at eleven million on advertising rates: *Woman's Own*—British magazine with readership estimated at six million on advertising rates; *Claire Rayner's Casebook*—BBC television programme with audience of approximately three million (official BBC figures); frequent appearances on radio and television discussing medical and social items, all of which generate letters asking for help and information. Volume of mail varies from week to week but average annual total is approximately 50 000.
4. Preston, N. W. Whooping cough immunisation; fact and fiction. *Publ Hlth (Lond)* 1980; 350–355.

Ethical Dilemmas in Health Promotion
Edited by S. Doxiadis

CHAPTER 18

Conclusions

SPYROS DOXIADIS

> 'It is a mark of the trained mind never to expect more precision in the treatment of any subject than the nature of that subject permits.' (Aristotle Ethics. Book one.)

In this last chapter, I wish to record some personal thoughts arising out of the preceding sections, of my contact and discussions with the other authors and of my numerous meetings with the members of the editorial committee to whom I wish to express here again my warm thanks for their hard work and friendly cooperation.

The first conclusion is that our initiative to undertake this long-term project and to ask for support from various agencies and individuals was justified indeed. There are today very important ethical issues and moral dilemmas in the field of health promotion and of disease prevention and these problems need to be studied and discussed. This is urgent because many of the problems have become evident only in recent years and they have not therefore been adequately and extensively discussed. Thus to most people they are unknown but the developments out of which they arise affect the life of all citizens and of all countries. Their importance needs to be recognized not only by a small group of scientists but by the wider community, by the mass communication media and by the decision-makers. Even since we began our work, ethical issues have been coming into sharper focus.

These problems and the need for their exploration are not confined to the traditional health sciences, the principal one of which is medicine. Many other disciplines are involved. It was, therefore, necessary to draw into this field representatives of many other sciences and professions and this is exemplified by the professional composition of the authors of our book. Out of the 21, only 13 are medical doctors. The others represent philosophy, theology, the law, economics, political science and journalism. The contribution of some of these disciplines has rightly been accepted as necessary in discussion of the ethical problems of therapeutic medicine. It becomes however indispensable, as the following paragraphs show, when exploring the ethical issues that arise from the activities of promoting public and individual health and of preventing disease.

Our wish to stimulate as large a group of individuals as possible to think about these matters and our desire that this book is read by many people who had not had previous experience in this field in and out of the health professions, made necessary the inclusion of chapters which provide background knowledge and a general introduction to the subject of medical ethics on the one hand and preventive medicine on the other. Thus in Part A in Chapter 1 the reader can find a review of the development of medical ethics which ends with a plea for recognition of the discipline of words. The theme of words and definitions continues in Chapter 2. When examining problems of definition it becomes evident that medical ethics—or better, as suggested 'health care ethics'—cannot be confined within the limits of medicine. This is more acutely so, as mentioned in the Introduction, in the field of preventive medicine and of health promotion which have to consider and be influenced by many social, cultural, political, economic and legal factors outside traditional medicine. In the same chapter a brief but succinct definition is given of the terms central to the critical analysis of medical ethics, such as personal freedom, common good, autonomy, paternalism, education, intervention.

In Chapter 3 a philosophical analysis is presented on the relationship between ethics and medical ethics. It is stressed that questions on the whole of medicine as a human activity, on its ultimate aims, on its interaction with other individual and social functions cannot be answered within medicine itself. These questions have to be answered by discussion and cooperation with other disciplines with an indispensable contribution from philosophy.

Chapter 4 describes and analyses the origins of public health and preventive medicine in modern times. In Chapter 5, the last chapter of the first part of the book, a description is given of the various models of disease causation and therefore of disease prevention as they have developed in recent times. The various obstacles to disease prevention are described so that the reader understands better the ethical and moral problems that can arise in the practice of preventive medicine.

Part B of the book contains six chapters which describe and analyse the general ethical problems in trying to improve public health. The central issue around which all questions revolve is the conflict of responsibilities, duties and rights between the state and the citizen, between the common good and the interest of the individual. It is obvious that some of these conflicts, especially perhaps those caused by scarcity of resources or by ignorance, may be satisfactorily resolved. This may take time but at least in theory, resolution is possible. There are other fields of conflict, however, in which solutions are not possible and this dilemma is examined in Chapter 6. We have to accept that there are situations and cases in which conflict is inevitable. It is not possible that one of the two parties, the state or the individual, will be the absolute winner. Complete sovereignty of the state (over the individual) or complete freedom of the individual are not possible in the modern complicated democratic society. Thus we have to accept that our efforts should aim not at the resolution or perfect solution but at the minimization of conflict between the efforts of the state for the common good and the struggle of the individual for his autonomy.

The question of state paternalism is another central ethical issue (Chapter 7). To what extent and in what circumstances is it justified? Respect for the absolute autonomy of the individual is impossible in the modern state. We have come not only to accept but to consider it an important duty of the community to provide collective goods which no individual can obtain for himself, beginning with clean water and sewage in the nineteenth century and progressing to the antipollution measures in the twentieth. To what extent, however, is state paternalism justified when it extends its activities into the life and life-style of the individual? Clear-cut limits to state paternalism are difficult, if not impossible, to define. In each case under discussion we have to consider many factors. One which should not be ignored is the psychological benefit of the citizen who by accepting public health measures is also encouraged to think more of his own life-style and health. He may be further influenced to accept group activities as promoting general welfare and this attitude may also make him accept the necessity of restricting his liberty to act in order to attain wider welfare and common goods. Absolute antipaternalism may also lead eventually to more restrictions of individual liberty by forcing the state and the community to adopt very restrictive measures.

Furthermore if we accept the absolute freedom and ability of the individual to regulate his own life we end with the concept of victim blaming. This leads us to forget that personal choices cannot be absolutely free from the influence of other factors. Advertisements, social and economic status, addiction are all factors that restrict absolute freedom. For example, the heavy smoker who has been subjected since childhood to constant brainwashing from cigarette advertisements, from peer pressure and from the negative effect of living with smoking parents cannot be held entirely responsible for his habit and be made to bear all the cost of treatment for any illnesses resulting from smoking. In this case intervention of the state to restrict or totally prohibit cigarette advertisements, since it is impossible to eliminate the other two factors, is morally justified. A balance of measures is therefore necessary, but a moderate degree of state paternalism is inevitable.

Whether it is possible or desirable to regulate by law all these aspects, including individual behaviour, is examined in Chapter 8. This has become an important question because in recent years legislation is entering the field of health promotion and therefore may also intrude into the life-style of individuals. This may lead to undesirable restrictions and constant awareness of this danger is necessary. It is further necessary through research and discussion to define the ethically acceptable limits of such intervention and to draw the line between regulatory, incentive and educative measures.

Education and behaviour control are not, however, without their own moral dilemmas which are described in Chapter 9. They have always existed from primitive societies to the present day. Every community tries to educate its young consciously or unconsciously so that they adopt desirable life habits and avoid what that community at that particular time considers as undesirable or injurious. Educative measures are today more effective and therefore they give more power to the state or groups or individuals which may impose them. This is another risk to personal autonomy and liberty of action. Such measures and especially those addressed to the young should not therefore be imposed before information is provided to the public and before their reactions and their wishes are ascertained. This becomes even more necessary when messages of health education do not simply provide factual information based on scientific knowledge but try to influence behaviour relying on value judgments.

Chapter 10 looks at the economic factors which have already entered in a very determined way into therapeutic medicine because of the rapidly rising cost of modern medical technology. They are, however, much more important in planning projects of health promotion and disease prevention because, since these projects are addressed to whole populations, they are much more expensive. And while in theory definition of targets and priorities should come first and economic considerations second, in practice there is often a continuous two-way interaction and a parallel consideration of both targets and the economic means to achieve them. Thus economists should be from the beginning part of the multidisciplinary team in planning large-scale projects and economic analysis must play an ever-increasing role in studying effectiveness and efficiency of all acts in both the clinical and the public health fields. Modern western society in its attempts to promote public and individual health for the common good, is inevitably restricted by economic factors. The discipline of economics should not, however, dictate the final objectives or impose a rigid plan, because priorities in the field of health should inevitably be defined by the health sciences and finally approved by the citizens through democratic procedures.

Part B ends with a chapter on occupational health and risks and the ethical imperative in preventive medicine to try to identify those risks and reduce their magnitude.

In the final part of the book some specific ethical issues are analysed. These issues are generated by practical public health problems which confront those involved in and responsible for the day-to-day planning and implementing of policies and programmes of public health (Chapters 12, 13, 14 and 15). The section continues with a chapter on the methodological aspects of ethical control in practice (Chapter 16) and ends with Chapter 17 in which the important contribution of the mass communication media in educating the public and the media's subsequent moral responsibilities are examined. A proposal is made on how to avoid the common errors and misunderstandings which still all too often arise between those in the media and those involved in health care.

So what should our recommendations be? I think the first and most important point is *to increase the awareness of all those responsible for making and implementing decisions in health promotion and disease prevention as to the existence of serious moral and ethical problems in these activities.* There are signs that this is beginning to happen. We should therefore encourage and extend at all levels discussion of the relevant ethical issues.

We should try to make everyone realize the great complexity of these problems. We physicians and other health professionals must not restrict the discussion to our own disciplines. The complexity of the problems and the impact of any decisions on the lives of many people make it imperative to invite the interest and cooperation of decision-makers and scientists from other disciplines.

And then *we have to inform the wider public.* In matters so relevant to the life and health of whole populations and likely to influence future generations, any kind of monopoly of decisions either by the state or by the health professions is to be condemned. Values differ from society to society and they may change as so many other things rapidly change in our times. We cannot afford to be dogmatic in our ideas or rigid in our decisions. A continuous exchange of ideas on attitudes, desires and expectations of the wider public on the one hand, and of knowledge and decisions of the experts and the decision-makers on the other, is essential in order to promote the health of all citizens and at the same time to respect the autonomy of the individual. For this, new and special arrangements are necessary. Methods and mechanisms will have to be instituted in the form of advisory agencies, of committees of experts, of representative bodies to inform, to discuss, to advise.

The discussion and the exploration of these issues should never stop. New problems will always arise and what is today considered an innocent and effective public health measure may be found tomorrow to be injurious for some individuals or for a whole community. This leads us to stress a second recommendation; *the need for further research.* On the one hand we need to know much more about the efficiency and the effectiveness of public health measures and on the other hand about the magnitude of risks of various factors or occurrences in our life. Only by such knowledge shall we be able to take more just decisions. But research is also needed to learn more about the values, attitudes, desires and expectations of the populations which the decisions we study and contemplate will affect.

All this work is not easy. Obstacles are many and obstruction and resistance from ignorance, from bias, or from political or economic interests are likely to be encountered in every case and at every stage. Without complaints or discouragement we should adopt a pragmatic approach trying in each case to combine the common good with the protection of the rights of the individual. Our task in this book has been to attempt to bring into focus some of the ethical dilemmas we face in preventive medicine and health promotion today. These dilemmas will not disappear—they must be confronted and resolved in a continuing effort to improve public health.

Index